ABC of Clinical Haematology

Fourth Edition

EDITED BY

Drew Provan

Emeritus Reader in Autoimmune Haematology
Department of Haematology
Barts and The London School of Medicine and Dentistry
Queen Mary University of London
London
UK

WILEY Blackwell

BMJ|Books

Registered Office(s)
John Wiley & Sons, Inc., 111 River Street, Hoboken, NJ 07030, USA
John Wiley & Sons Ltd, The Atrium, Southern Gate, Chichester, West Sussex, PO19 8SQ, UK

Editorial Office
9600 Garsington Road, Oxford, OX4 2DQ, UK

For details of our global editorial offices, customer services, and more information about Wiley products visit us at www.wiley.com.

Wiley also publishes its books in a variety of electronic formats and by print-on-demand. Some content that appears in standard print versions of this book may not be available in other formats.

Library of Congress Cataloging-in-Publication Data

Names: Provan, Drew, 1955– editor.
Title: ABC of clinical haematology / edited by Drew Provan.
Description: Fourth edition. | Hoboken, NJ : John Wiley & Sons, Inc., 2018. | Includes bibliographical
    references and index. |
Identifiers: LCCN 2017055360 (print) | LCCN 2017056756 (ebook) | ISBN 9781118892473 (pdf) |
    ISBN 9781118892480 (epub) | ISBN 9781118892343 (pbk.)
Subjects: | MESH: Hematologic Diseases–diagnosis | Hematologic Diseases–therapy |
    Hematologic Diseases–physiopathology
Classification: LCC RC633 (ebook) | LCC RC633 (print) | NLM WH 120 | DDC 616.1/5–dc23
LC record available at https://lccn.loc.gov/2017055360

Cover Design: Wiley
Cover Image: © Science Photo Library - STEVE GSCHMEISSNER./Gettyimages

Set in 9.25/12pt Minion by SPi Global, Pondicherry, India
Printed and bound in Singapore by Markono Print Media Pte Ltd

10 9 8 7 6 5 4 3 2 1

Contents

Contributors

Katharine Bailey
Haematology, Cancer Institute, UCL, Royal Free Campus, London, UK

Catherine Booth
Specialist Registrar in Haematology, Barts and the London NHS Trust, London, UK

Richard Burt
Haematology, Cancer Institute, UCL, Royal Free Campus, London, UK

Tom Butler
Department of Clinical Haematology, Barts Health NHS Trust, Pathology & Pharmacy Building, Royal London Hospital, London, UK

Jenny L. Byrne
Nottingham University Hospitals NHS Trust, Nottingham, UK

Jamie Cavenagh
Consultant Haematologist, Department of Haemato-Oncology, St Bartholomew's Hospital, West Smithfield, London, UK

John de Vos
Consultant Haematologist, Royal Surrey County Hospital NHS Foundation Trust, Guildford, UK

Robin Dowse
Senior Specialist Registrar, Haematological Medicine, King's College Hospital NHS Foundation Trust, Hambleden Wing, London, UK

Adele K. Fielding
Haematology, Cancer Institute, UCL, Royal Free Campus, London, UK

Anna L. Godfrey
Consultant Haematologist, Department of Haematology, Cambridge University Hospitals NHS Foundation Trust, Cambridge, UK

Anthony R. Green
Director, Wellcome Trust/MRC Cambridge Stem Cell Institute, University of Cambridge;
Department of Haematology, University of Cambridge, Cambridge, UK

Sandra Hassan
Consultant Haematologist, Queen's Hospital, BHR NHS Trust, Romford, UK

Catherine Hockings
Department of Haematology, University College London Hospitals NHS Foundation Trust, London, UK

Victor Hoffbrand
Emeritus Professor of Haematology, University College London, London, UK

David M. Keeling
Consultant Haematologist, Oxford University Hospitals, Oxford Haemophilia & Thrombosis Centre, Churchill Hospital, Oxford, UK

R. J. Liesner
Director Haemophilia CCC, Great Ormond Street Hospital, London, UK

Christopher McNamara
Department of Haematology, University College London Hospitals NHS Foundation Trust, London, UK

Ghulam J. Mufti
Professor of Haemato-oncology & Head of Department, Haematological Medicine, King's College Hospital NHS Foundation Trust, Hambleden Wing, London, UK

Jim Murray
Haematology – University Hospitals Birmingham NHS Foundation Trust, Queen Elizabeth Hospital, Queen Elizabeth Medical Centre, Birmingham, UK

Adrian C. Newland
Barts and the London Medical School, Queen Mary University of London; Department of Clinical Haematology, Barts Health NHS Trust, Pathology & Pharmacy Building, Royal London Hospital, London, UK

Igor Novitzky-Basso
Stem Cell Laboratory Medical Director, Queen Elizabeth University Hospital Glasgow, NHS Greater Glasgow and Clyde, Glasgow, UK

Drew Provan
Emeritus Reader in Autoimmune Haematology, Department of Haematology, Barts and The London School of Medicine and Dentistry, Queen Mary University of London, London, UK

Marie A. Scully

Department of Haematology, University College London Hospitals NHS Trust, Cardiometabolic Programme-NIHR UCLH/UCL BRC, London, UK

Julia Sikorska

Specialist Registrar in Haematology, Royal Surrey County Hospital NHS Foundation Trust, Guildford, UK

George S. Vassiliou

Group Leader and Consultant Haematologist, Wellcome Trust Sanger Institute, Wellcome Genome Campus, Hinxton; Wellcome Trust/MRC Cambridge Stem Cell Institute, University of Cambridge, Cambridge, UK

David J. Weatherall

Regius Professor of Medicine Emeritus, MRC Weatherall Institute of Molecular Medicine, University of Oxford, Headington, Oxford, UK

CHAPTER 1

Iron-Deficiency Anaemia

Drew Provan[1] and Catherine Booth[2]

[1] Department of Haematology, Barts and The London School of Medicine and Dentistry,
Queen Mary University of London, London, UK
[2] Barts and the London NHS Trust, London, UK

OVERVIEW

- Iron deficiency is the commonest cause of anaemia worldwide and is frequently seen in general practice.
- The anaemia of iron deficiency is caused by defective synthesis of haemoglobin, resulting in red cells that are smaller than normal (microcytic) and contain reduced amounts of haemoglobin (hypochromic).

Iron metabolism

Iron has a pivotal role in many metabolic processes, and the average adult contains 3–5 g of iron, of which two-thirds is in the oxygen-carrying molecule haemoglobin.

A normal Western diet provides about 15 mg of iron daily, of which 5–10% is absorbed (~1 mg), principally in the duodenum and upper jejunum, where the acidic conditions help the absorption of iron in the ferrous form. Absorption is helped by the presence of other reducing substances, such as hydrochloric acid and ascorbic acid. The body has the capacity to increase its iron absorption in the face of increased demand – for example, in pregnancy, lactation, growth spurts and iron deficiency (Box 1.1).

Once absorbed from the bowel, iron is transported across the mucosal cell to the blood, where it is carried by the protein transferrin to developing red cells in the bone marrow. Iron stores comprise ferritin, a labile and readily accessible source of iron, and haemosiderin, an insoluble form found predominantly in macrophages.

About 1 mg of iron a day is lost from the body in urine, faeces, sweat and cells shed from the skin and gastrointestinal tract. Menstrual losses of an additional 20 mg a month, and the increased requirements of pregnancy (500–1000 mg) contribute to the higher incidence of iron deficiency in women of reproductive age (Table 1.1, Box 1.2).

Box 1.1 **Risk factors for development of iron deficiency.**

- **Age:** infants (especially if history of prematurity); adolescents; premenopausal women; old age
- **Gender:** increased risk in women
- **Reproduction:** pregnancy, breast feeding
- **Travel/country of origin:** parasites (e.g. hookworm, schistosoma)
- **Gastrointestinal pathology:** appetite or weight changes; changes in bowel habit; bleeding from rectum/melaena; gastric or bowel surgery
- **Drug history:** especially aspirin and non-steroidal anti-inflammatories
- **Social history:** diet, especially vegetarianism, age of weaning of infants

Clinical features of iron deficiency

The symptoms accompanying iron deficiency depend on how rapidly the anaemia develops. In cases of chronic, slow blood loss, the body adapts to the increasing anaemia, and patients can often tolerate extremely low concentrations of haemoglobin (e.g. <70 g/L) with remarkably few symptoms. Most patients complain of increasing lethargy and dyspnoea. More unusual symptoms are headaches, tinnitus, taste disturbance and restless leg syndrome. Pica (a desire to eat non-food substances) and, most characteristically, pagophagia (abnormal consumption of ice) are uncommon but well described, resolving promptly with iron replacement. In children, chronic iron-deficiency anaemia can lead to impaired psychomotor and cognitive development.

On examination, several skin, nail and other epithelial changes may be seen in chronic iron deficiency. Atrophy of the skin occurs in about a third of patients, and (rarely nowadays) nail changes such as

Table 1.1 Daily dietary iron requirements.

Male	1 mg
Adolescence	2–3 mg
Female (reproductive age)	2–3 mg
Pregnancy	3–4 mg
Infancy	1 mg
Maximum bioavailability from normal diet	~4 mg

Box 1.2 Causes of iron-deficiency anaemia.

Most iron-deficiency anaemia is the result of blood loss, especially in affluent countries.

Reproductive system
- Menorrhagia

Gastrointestinal tract

Bleeding
- Oesophagitis
- Oesophageal varices
- Hiatus hernia (ulcerated)
- Peptic ulcer
- Inflammatory bowel disease
- Haemorrhoids (rarely)
- Carcinoma: stomach, colorectal
- Angiodysplasia
- Hereditary haemorrhagic telangiectasia (rare)
- Hookworm infection – commonest cause of iron deficiency worldwide

Malabsorption
- Coeliac disease
- Atrophic gastritis (also may result *from* iron deficiency)
- Infection: *Helicobacter pylori*, tropical sprue
- Post-surgical: gastric bypass, small bowel resection

Renal tract
- Haematuria – *Schistosoma haematobium* infection
- Intravascular haemolysis with renal haemosiderin excretion

Physiological (increased demand)
- Growth spurts (especially in premature infants)
- Pregnancy, lactation

Dietary
- Vegans
- Elderly
- Infants under 12 months fed predominantly on cow's milk

Other
- Iatrogenic: multiple blood sampling (especially premature infants)
- Patients with chronic renal failure undergoing haemodialysis and receiving erythropoietin

koilonychia (spoon-shaped nails) may result in brittle, flattened nails (Figure 1.1). Patients may also complain of angular stomatitis, in which painful cracks appear at the angle of the mouth, sometimes accompanied by glossitis. Although uncommon, oesophageal and pharyngeal webs can be a feature of iron-deficiency anaemia (consider this in middle-aged women presenting with dysphagia).

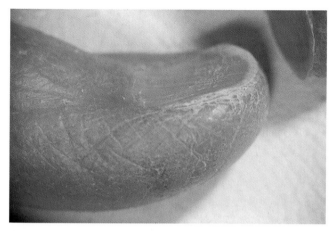

Figure 1.1 Nail changes in iron-deficiency anaemia (koilonychia).

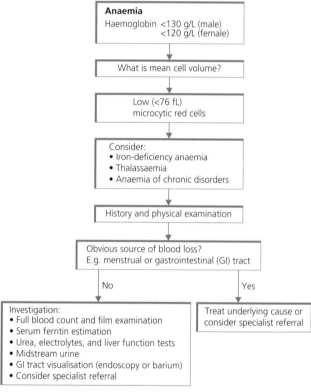

Figure 1.2 Diagnosis and investigation of iron-deficiency anaemia.

These changes are believed to be due to a reduction in the iron-containing enzymes in the epithelium and gastrointestinal tract. Few of these epithelial changes are seen in modern practice, and are of limited diagnostic value.

Tachycardia and cardiac failure may occur with severe anaemia irrespective of cause, and in such cases prompt remedial action should be taken.

When iron deficiency is confirmed, a full clinical history including leading questions on possible gastrointestinal blood loss or malabsorption (e.g. as in coeliac disease) should be obtained. Menstrual losses should be assessed, and the importance of dietary factors and regular blood donation should not be overlooked (Figure 1.2).

ABC of
Clinical Haematology

Fourth Edition

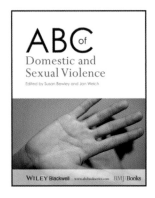
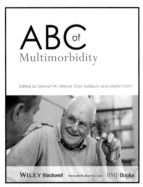
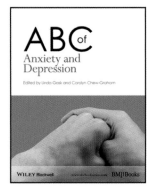
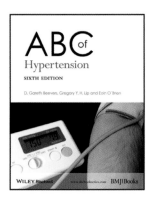
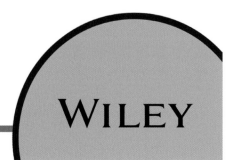

Diet alone is seldom the sole cause for iron-deficiency anaemia in adults in Britain except when it prevents an adequate response to a physiological challenge – as in pregnancy, for example. In children, by contrast, diet is a key factor, particularly in infants slow to wean (e.g. by 6 months) or those fed cow's milk (which has low iron content and poor bioavailability) before 12 months.

Laboratory investigations

A full blood count and film should be assessed (Box 1.3). These will confirm the anaemia, and recognising the indices of iron deficiency is usually straightforward – reduced haemoglobin concentration, reduced mean cell volume (MCV), reduced mean cell haemoglobin (MCH), reduced mean cell haemoglobin concentration (MCHC). Some modern analysers will determine the percentage of hypochromic red cells, which may be high before the anaemia develops (it is worth noting that a reduction in haemoglobin concentration is a *late* feature of iron deficiency – the first change being an increase in the red cell distribution width). There may be a reactive thrombocytosis. The blood film shows microcytic hypochromic red cells, pencil cells and occasional target cells (Table 1.2, Figure 1.3).

Hypochromic anaemia occurs in other disorders, such as anaemia of chronic disorders and sideroblastic anaemias and in globin synthesis disorders, such as thalassaemia (Table 1.3). Difficulties in diagnosis arise when more than one type of anaemia is present – for example, iron deficiency and folate deficiency in malabsorption, in a population where thalassaemia is present, or in pregnancy, when the interpretation of red cell indices may be difficult. To help to

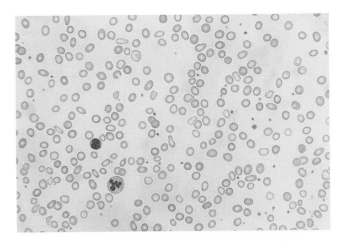

Figure 1.3 Blood film showing changes of iron-deficiency anaemia.

differentiate the type, further haematinic assays are used. Iron levels alone are unhelpful due to wide diurnal variation and poor sensitivity. Low levels in combination with a raised total iron binding capacity (or transferrin) – often expressed as a reduced transferrin saturation – are more suggestive.

The haematinic measure of choice is serum ferritin, reduced levels being highly specific for iron deficiency. However, its sensitivity is limited, in part because, as an acute-phase protein, the concentration may be normal or even raised in inflammatory or malignant disease. A prime example of this is found in rheumatoid disease, in which active disease may result in a spuriously raised serum ferritin concentration masking an underlying iron deficiency caused by gastrointestinal bleeding after non-steroidal analgesic treatment. There may also be confusion in liver disease, as the liver contains stores of ferritin that are released after hepatocellular damage, leading to raised serum ferritin concentrations. In cases where ferritin estimation is likely to be misleading, the soluble transferrin receptor (sTfR) assay may aid the diagnosis. Transferrin receptors are found on the surface of red cells in greater numbers in iron deficiency; a proportion of receptors are shed into the plasma and can be measured. sTfR is not increased in inflammatory disorders, and hence can help differentiate between anaemia due to inflammation from iron deficiency. Zinc protoporphyrin (ZPP) is another alternative assay. Levels rise in iron deficiency as zinc takes the place of iron in the final stage of haem synthesis. However, ZPP is elevated (albeit to a lesser degree) whenever there is impaired ability to utilise iron, which includes chronic inflammatory states and thalassaemia.

Diagnostic bone marrow sampling is seldom performed in simple iron deficiency, but if the diagnosis is in doubt a marrow aspirate may be carried out to demonstrate absent bone marrow stores.

When iron deficiency has been diagnosed, the underlying cause should be investigated and treated. Often the history will indicate the likely source of bleeding – for example, menstrual blood loss or gastrointestinal bleeding. If there is no obvious cause, further investigation generally depends on the age and sex of the patient. Coeliac serology should be sent even if the patient has no gastrointestinal symptoms, as coeliac disease may present with iron deficiency alone. In male patients and postmenopausal women, possible gastrointestinal blood loss is investigated by visualisation

---

Box 1.3 Investigations in iron-deficiency anaemia.

- Full clinical history and physical examination
- Full blood count and blood film examination
- Haematinic assays (serum ferritin, vitamin B_{12} folate)
- Percentage hypochromic red cells and soluble transferrin receptor assay (if available)
- Urea and electrolytes, liver function tests
- Fibre-optic and/or barium studies of gastrointestinal tract
- Pelvic ultrasound (females, if indicated)

Table 1.2 Diagnosis of iron-deficiency anaemia (normal values in parentheses).

Reduced haemoglobin	Men <130 g/L, women <120 g/L
Reduced MCV	<76 fL (76–95 fL)
Reduced MCH	29.5±2.5 pg (27.0–32.0 pg)
Reduced MCHC	32.5±2.5 g/dL (32.0–36.0 g/dL)
Blood film	Microcytic hypochromic red cells with pencil cells and target cells
Reduced serum ferritin[a]	<15 µg/L (men and women) <15 µg/L (premenopausal) <10 µg/L
Elevated percentage of hypochromic red cells (>2%)	
Elevated soluble transferrin receptor level	
Elevated zinc protoporphyrin	

[a] Check with local laboratory for reference ranges.

Table 1.3 Characteristics of anaemia associated with other disorders.

	Iron deficiency	Chronic disorders	Thalassaemia trait (α or β)	Sideroblastic anaemia
Degree of anaemia	Any	Seldom <90 g/L	Mild	Any
MCV	↓	N or ↓	↓↓	N or ↓ or ↑
Serum ferritin	↓	N or ↑	N	↑
Soluble transferrin receptor assay	↑	N	↑	N
Zinc protoporphyrin	↑↑	↑	↑	↑ or ↑↑
Marrow iron	Absent	Present	Present	Present

N: normal.

of the gastrointestinal tract via endoscopy (upper and lower). It may occasionally be necessary to proceed to radiographic or wireless capsule investigation of the small bowel if endoscopies are normal and clinical suspicion remains high.

Management

Effective management of iron deficiency relies on (a) the appropriate management of the underlying cause (e.g. gastrointestinal or menstrual blood loss) and (b) iron replacement therapy.

Oral iron replacement therapy with gradual replenishment of iron stores and restoration of haemoglobin is the preferred treatment (Table 1.4, Figure 1.4). Oral ferrous salts are the treatment of choice (ferric salts are less well absorbed) and usually take the form of ferrous sulphate 200 mg three times daily (providing 65 mg×3 = 195 mg elemental iron per day). Alternative preparations include ferrous gluconate and ferrous fumarate. All three compounds, however, are associated with a high incidence of side effects, including nausea, constipation and diarrhoea. These side effects may be reduced by taking the tablets after meals, but even

Table 1.4 Elemental iron content of various oral iron preparations.

Preparation	Amount (mg)	Ferrous iron (mg)
Ferrous sulphate	200	65
Ferrous gluconate	300	35
Ferrous fumarate	210	65–70

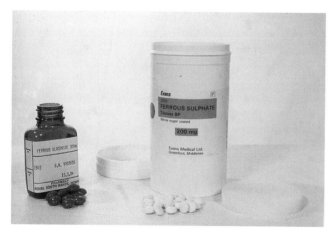

Figure 1.4 Oral iron replacement therapy.

milder symptoms account for poor compliance with oral iron supplementation. These lower gastrointestinal symptoms are not always dose related. Modified-release preparations have been developed to reduce side effects but in practice prove expensive and often release the iron beyond the sites of optimal absorption.

Effective iron replacement therapy should result in a rise in haemoglobin concentration of around 1 g/L per day (about 20 g/L every 3 weeks), with a response seen within 5–7 days, but this varies from patient to patient. Once the haemoglobin concentration is within the normal range, iron replacement should continue for 3 months to replenish the iron stores.

Failure to respond to oral iron therapy

The main reason for failure to respond to oral iron therapy is poor compliance. However, if the losses (e.g. bleeding) exceed the amount of iron absorbed daily, the haemoglobin concentration will not rise as expected; this will also be the case in combined deficiency states.

The presence of underlying inflammation or malignancy may also lead to a poor response to therapy. Occasionally, malabsorption of iron, such as that seen in coeliac disease, may lead to a failure to respond. High levels of dietary phytates (bran, oats, rye), polyphenols (tea) and calcium may impair absorption of iron if taken together. Finally, an incorrect diagnosis of iron-deficiency anaemia should be considered in patients who fail to respond adequately to iron replacement therapy.

Intravenous iron preparations

Parenteral iron may be used when the patient cannot tolerate oral supplements – for example, when patients have severe gastrointestinal side effects or if the losses exceed the daily amount that can be absorbed orally. Patients on renal dialysis receiving erythropoietin also routinely require intravenous iron.

Intravenous iron should be given under strict medical supervision (e.g. on a haematology day unit) due to the risk of anaphylaxis or other reactions. Full resuscitation facilities must be available, and a test dose is recommended before administration of the full dose. Preparations include Venofer and Ferinject, given in several divided doses, and Cosmofer and Monofer, which can be administered as a single total dose infusion (Box 1.4).

The dose is based on the estimated iron deficit, calculated using the Ganzoni formula (Box 1.5). In practice, quick reference tables are available giving the dose for the patient's weight and target versus actual haemoglobin level.

Box 1.4 **Intravenous iron preparations.**

Compound	Trade name	Elemental iron concentration (mg/mL)	Administration
Iron hydroxide dextran	CosmoFer	50	Total dose infusion (max. 20 mg iron/kg body weight)
Iron isomaltoside	Monofer	100	Total dose infusion (max. 20 mg iron/kg body weight)
Iron sucrose	Venofer	20	Max. dose 200 mg iron, up to three times per week
Ferric carboxymaltose	Ferinject	50	Max. dose 1000 mg iron, once per week

Box 1.5 **Iron dose calculation.**

$$\text{Total dose} = \text{Body weight(kg)} \times [\text{Target Hb} + \text{Actual Hb}](\text{g/L}) \times 0.24 + 500 \text{ mg for iron stores}$$

where 0.24 is the percentage blood volume by weight (7%) × iron content of haemoglobin (Hb, 0.34%) × 1000 (grams to milligrams conversion).

The rise in haemoglobin concentration is no faster with parenteral iron preparations than with oral iron therapy.

Alternative treatments

Blood transfusion is not indicated unless the patient has decompensated due to a drop in haemoglobin concentration and needs a more rapid rise in haemoglobin – for example, in cases of worsening angina or severe coexisting pulmonary disease. In cases of iron deficiency with serious ongoing acute bleeding, blood transfusion may be required.

Prevention

When absorption from the diet is likely to be matched or exceeded by losses, extra sources of iron should be considered – for example, prophylactic iron supplements in pregnancy, for premature infants or after gastrectomy, or encouragement of breast feeding or use of formula milk rather than cow's milk during the first year of life.

Acknowledgements

Dr AG Smith and Dr A Amos provided the photographic material.

Further reading

Baer AN, Dessypris EN and Krantz SB (1990) The pathogenesis of anemia in rheumatoid arthritis: a clinical and laboratory analysis. *Seminars in Arthritis and Rheumatism*, **19**(4), 209–223.

Beguin Y (2003) Soluble transferrin receptor for the evaluation of erythropoiesis and iron status. *Clinica Chimica Acta*, **329**(1–2), 9–22.

Cook JD, Skikne BS and Baynes RD (1994) Iron deficiency: the global perspective. *Advances in Experimental Medicine and Biology*, **356**, 219–228.

Cook JD (2005) Diagnosis and management of iron-deficiency anaemia. *Best Practice & Research Clinical Haematology*, **18**(2), 319–332.

DeMaeyer E and Adiels-Tegman M (1985) The prevalence of anaemia in the world. *World Health Statistics Quarterly*, **38**(3), 302–316.

Demir A, Yarali N, Fisgin T, *et al.* (2004) Serum transferrin receptor levels in beta-thalassemia trait. *Journal of Tropical Pediatrics*, **50**(6), 369–371.

Electronic Medicines Compendium (eMC+) (n.d.) Summaries of product characteristics (SPCs) of licensed medicines. www.medicines.org.uk (accessed 3 September 2017).

Ferguson BJ, Skikne BS, Simpson KM, *et al.* (1992) Serum transferrin receptor distinguishes the anemia of chronic disease from iron deficiency anemia. *Journal of Laboratory and Clinical Medicine*, **119**(4), 385–390.

Lozoff B, De Andraca I, Castillo M, *et al.* (2003) Behavioral and developmental effects of preventing iron-deficiency anemia in healthy full-term infants. *Pediatrics*, **112**(4), 846–854.

McIntyre AS and Long RG (1993) Prospective survey of investigations in outpatients referred with iron deficiency anaemia. *Gut*, **34**(8), 1102–1107.

Provan D (1999) Mechanisms and management of iron deficiency anaemia. *British Journal of Haematology*, **105**(Suppl 1), 19–26.

Punnonen K, Irjala K and Rajamaki A (1997) Serum transferrin receptor and its ratio to serum ferritin in the diagnosis of iron deficiency. *Blood*, **89**(3), 1052–1057.

Rockey DC and Cello JP (1993) Evaluation of the gastrointestinal tract in patients with iron-deficiency anemia. *New England Journal of Medicine*, **329**(23), 1691–1695.

Windsor CW and Collis JL (1967) Anaemia and hiatus hernia: experience in 450 patients. *Thorax*, **22**(1), 73–78.

CHAPTER 2

Macrocytic Anaemias

Victor Hoffbrand

University College London, London, UK

OVERVIEW

- Macrocytic red cells (mean cell volume >95 fL) may be associated with a megaloblastic or normoblastic bone marrow.
- Deficiencies of either vitamin B_{12} or folate lead to defective DNA synthesis, megaloblastic changes in the bone marrow and many other cells.
- The blood count indices and blood film features of B_{12} and folate deficiencies are identical and specific haematinic assays are required to differentiate between them.
- Pernicious anaemia (PA) is the commonest cause of B_{12} deficiency in the UK.
- Folate deficiency occurs in pregnancy, prematurity, chronic haemolysis gluten-induced enteropathy (coeliac disease) and other high cell turnover states.

Vitamin B_{12} deficiency may lead to progressive neuropathy even in the absence of anaemia. Macrocytosis is a rise in the mean cell volume (MCV) of the red cells above the normal range (in adults 80–95 fL). It is detected with a blood count, in which the MCV, as well as other red cell indices, is measured. The MCV is lower in children than in adults, with a normal mean of 70 fL at age 1 year, rising by about 1 fL each year until the child reaches adult volumes at puberty.

The causes of macrocytosis fall into two groups: (a) deficiency of vitamin B_{12} (cobalamin) or folate (or rarely abnormalities of their metabolism) in which the bone marrow is megaloblastic (Box 2.1), and (b) other causes, in which the bone marrow is usually normoblastic. In this chapter the two groups are considered separately. The reader is then taken through the steps to diagnose the cause of macrocytosis, and subsequently to manage it.

Megaloblastic bone marrow is exemplified by developing red blood cells that are larger than normal, with nuclei more immature than their cytoplasm. The underlying mechanism is defective DNA synthesis.

Deficiency of vitamin B_{12} (cobalamin) or folate

Vitamin B_{12} deficiency

The body's requirement for vitamin B_{12} (cobalamin, B_{12}) is about 1 µg daily. This is amply supplied by a normal Western diet (B_{12} content 10–30 µg daily) that includes animal products. Absorption of B_{12} is through the ileum, facilitated by intrinsic factor, which is secreted by the parietal cells of the stomach. Absorption by this mechanism is limited to 2–3 µg daily. Most of the B_{12} in plasma is bound to transcobalamin 1 (TC1, haptocorrin) and is metabolically 'dead', while a small fraction is attached to TC2 (transcobalamin), which nevertheless is the transport protein responsible for delivering B_{12} to marrow and all the other cells of the body.

In Britain, B_{12} deficiency is usually due to PA, which now accounts for up to 80% of all cases of megaloblastic anaemia. The incidence of the disease is 1:10 000 in northern Europe; the disease occurs in all races. The underlying mechanism is an autoimmune gastritis that results in achlorhydria and the absence of intrinsic factor. *Helicobacter pylori* may be an initiating factor for the gastritis but usually cannot be detected when PA develops. The incidence of PA peaks at age 60; the condition has a female:male incidence of 1.6:1.0 and is more common in those with early greying, blue eyes and blood group A, and in those with a family history of the disease or of diseases that may be associated with it – for example, vitiligo (Figure 2.1), myxoedema, Hashimoto's disease, Addison's disease of the adrenal gland and hypoparathyroidism.

Other causes of severe B_{12} deficiency are infrequent in Britain. B_{12} is only present in foods of animal origin, such as meat, fish, eggs, cheese and other dairy products. It is absent from fruit, vegetables and nuts. Veganism is an unusual cause of severe deficiency, as most vegetarians and vegans include some B_{12} in their diet. Moreover, unlike in PA, the enterohepatic circulation for B_{12} is intact in vegans, so B_{12} in bile is reabsorbed and stores are conserved. Gastric resection and intestinal causes of malabsorption of B_{12} are less common causes of the deficiency than PA is in the UK.

ABC of Clinical Haematology, Fourth Edition. Edited by Drew Provan.
© 2018 John Wiley & Sons Ltd. Published 2018 by John Wiley & Sons Ltd.

Box 2.1 **Causes of megaloblastic anaemia.**

Diet
- Vitamin B_{12} deficiency: veganism
- Folate deficiency: poor-quality diet, old age, poverty, synthetic diet without added folic acid, goats' milk

Malabsorption
- Gastric causes of vitamin B_{12} deficiency: pernicious anaemia (PA), congenital intrinsic factor deficiency or abnormality, gastrectomy
- Intestinal causes of vitamin B_{12} deficiency: stagnant loop, congenital selective malabsorption, ileal resection, Crohn's disease
- Intestinal causes of folate deficiency: gluten-induced enteropathy (coeliac disease), tropical sprue, jejunal resection

Increased cell turnover
- Folate deficiency: pregnancy, prematurity, chronic haemolytic anaemia (such as sickle cell anaemia), extensive inflammatory and malignant diseases

Renal loss
- Folate deficiency: congestive cardiac failure, dialysis

Drugs
- Folate deficiency: anticonvulsants, sulphasalazine

Defects of vitamin B_{12} metabolism (e.g. transcobalamin (TC2) deficiency, nitrous oxide anaesthesia) or of folate metabolism (such as methotrexate treatment) or rare inherited defects of DNA synthesis may all cause megaloblastic anaemia.

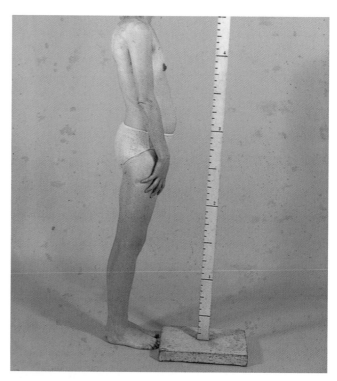

Figure 2.2 Patient with gluten-induced enteropathy (coeliac disease): underweight and low stature.

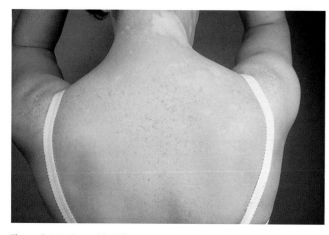

Figure 2.1 Patient with vitiligo on neck and back.

Mild degrees of B_{12} deficiency shown by a low serum B_{12} without macrocytosis are more frequent. They may be due to malabsorption of food B_{12} due to atrophic gastritis and achlorhydria with failure of release by pepsin and acid of food B_{12} from its protein binding. This occurs slightly more frequently in the elderly and in those with *H. pylori* infection than in controls. Mild B_{12} deficiency may also occur in severe pancreatitis, in gluten-induced enteropathy and due to prolonged therapy with proton pump inhibitors, in HIV infection and following stem cell transplantation with chronic graft versus host disease affecting the ileum. Metformin lowers serum TC1, and so serum B_{12}, but this would be metabolically neutral since TC1 binds B_{12} but is not involved in transport of B_{12} into cells for which

TC2 is responsible. Rarely, genetically low serum TC1 levels account for low serum B_{12} levels, but again these are of no clinical importance.

Folate deficiency

The daily requirement for folate is 100–200 µg, and a normal mixed diet contains about 200–300 µg. Natural folates are largely in the polyglutamate form, and these are absorbed through the upper small intestine after deconjugation and conversion to the monoglutamate, 5-methyltetrahydrofolate.

Body stores are sufficient for only about 4 months. Folate deficiency may arise because of inadequate dietary intake, malabsorption (especially gluten-induced enteropathy; Figure 2.2) or excessive use, since proliferating cells degrade folate because of its incomplete recycling in its role as coenzyme in reactions involved in DNA synthesis. Deficiency in pregnancy may be due partly to inadequate diet, partly to transfer of folate to the fetus and partly to increased folate degradation.

Consequences of vitamin B_{12} or folate deficiencies
Megaloblastic anaemia

Clinical features include pallor and jaundice. The onset is gradual, and a severely anaemic patient may present in congestive heart failure or only when an infection supervenes. The blood film (Figure 2.3) shows *oval* macrocytes and hypersegmented neutrophil nuclei (with six or more lobes). In severe cases, the white cell count and platelet count also fall (pancytopenia). The bone marrow shows characteristic megaloblastic erythroblasts and giant metamyelocytes (granulocyte precursors). Biochemically, there is an

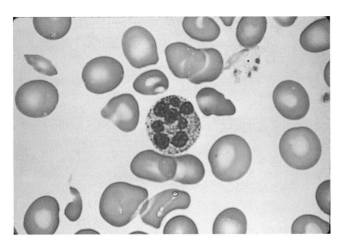

Figure 2.3 Blood film in vitamin B$_{12}$ deficiency showing macrocytic red cells and a hypersegmented neutrophil.

increase in plasma unconjugated bilirubin and serum lactic dehydrogenase, with, in severe cases, an absence of haptoglobins and presence in urine of haemosiderin. These changes, including jaundice, are due to increased destruction of red cell precursors, including haemoglobin, in the marrow (ineffective erythropoiesis).

Vitamin B$_{12}$ neuropathy
A minority of patients with severe B$_{12}$ deficiency, shown by a very low serum B$_{12}$ level, develop a neuropathy due to symmetrical damage to the peripheral nerves and posterior and lateral columns of the spinal cord, with the legs being more affected than the arms. Psychiatric abnormalities and visual disturbance may also occur. Men are more commonly affected than women. The neuropathy may occur in the absence of anaemia. Psychiatric changes may also occur in folate deficiency, but not the neuropathy. Cognitive deterioration has been ascribed to B$_{12}$ or folate deficiency, and the most recent trials of prophylaxis with B$_{12}$ and folic acid do suggest that these deficiencies may play a small role in some subjects.

Neural tube defects
Folic acid supplements in pregnancy have been shown to reduce the incidence of neural tube defects (spina bifida, encephalocoele and anencephaly) in the fetus and may also reduce the incidence of cleft palate and hare lip (Box 2.2). No clear relation exists, however, between the incidence of these defects and folate deficiency in the mother, although the lower the maternal red cell folate (and serum B$_{12}$) concentrations even within the normal range, the more likely neural tube defects are to occur in the fetus. An underlying mechanism in a minority of cases is a genetic defect in folate metabolism, a mutation in the enzyme 5,10-methylenetetrahydrofolate reductase.

Gonadal dysfunction
Deficiency of either B$_{12}$ or folate may cause sterility, which is reversible with appropriate vitamin supplementation.

Epithelial cell changes
Glossitis and other epithelial surfaces may show cytological abnormalities (Figure 2.4). This can lead to abnormalities in a cervical smear that may wrongly be ascribed to malignancy.

Box 2.2 **Preventing folate deficiency in pregnancy.**

- As prophylaxis against folate deficiency in pregnancy, daily doses of folic acid 400 µg are usual
- Larger doses are not recommended as they could theoretically 'mask' megaloblastic anaemia due to B$_{12}$ deficiency and thus allow B$_{12}$ neuropathy to develop
- As neural tube defects occur by the 28th day of pregnancy, it is advisable for a woman's daily folate intake to be increased by 400 µg/day at the time of conception
- The US Food and Drugs Administration announced in 1996 that specified grain products (including most enriched breads, flours, cornmeal, rice, noodles and macaroni) will be required to be fortified with folic acid to levels ranging from 0.43 to 1.5 µg per pound (453 g) of product. Fortification is now carried out in >70 countries and has been associated with a reduction in incidence of neural tube defects. Fortification of flour with folic acid has been under discussion in the UK for almost 20 years but has not been implemented because of, in this author's opinion, unwarranted fears that the low fortification doses of folic acid recommended may nevertheless lead to an increased incidence of B$_{12}$ neuropathy in the elderly.
- For mothers who have already had an infant with a neural tube defect, larger doses of folic acid (e.g. 5 mg daily) are recommended before and during subsequent pregnancy

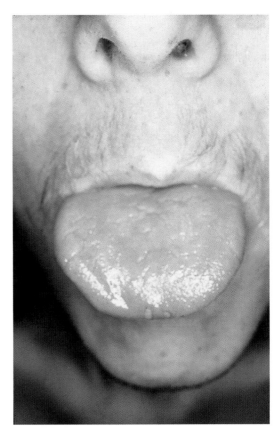

Figure 2.4 Glossitis due to vitamin B$_{12}$ deficiency.

Cardiovascular disease

Raised serum homocysteine concentrations have been associated with arterial obstruction (myocardial infarct, peripheral vascular disease or stroke) and venous thrombosis. Folic acid supplementation has not been found to reduce the risk of these cardiovascular diseases, except possibly a small reduction in incidence of stroke.

Other causes of macrocytosis

There are a number of other causes of macrocytosis (Box 2.3). The most common cause in Britain is alcohol. Small quantities of alcohol (e.g. two gin and tonics or half a bottle of wine a day) especially in women, may cause a rise of MCV to >100 fL, typically without anaemia or any detectable change in liver function.

The mechanism for the rise in MCV is uncertain, and there is no evidence that alone it is harmful, although it may provide a warning that alcohol consumption should not be increased and possibly be reduced. Because of the 120-day lifespan of red cells, it takes 3–4 months for the MCV to return to normal if alcohol consumption is stopped. In liver disease the red cell volume may rise due to excessive lipid deposition on red cell membranes, and the rise is particularly pronounced in liver disease caused by alcohol. A modest rise in MCV is found in severe thyroid deficiency.

Physiological causes of macrocytosis are pregnancy and the neonatal period. In other causes of macrocytosis, other haematological abnormalities are usually present – in myelodysplasia (a frequent cause of macrocytosis in elderly people) there are usually quantitative or qualitative changes in the white cells and platelets in the blood. In aplastic anaemia, pancytopenia is present; pure red cell aplasia may also cause macrocytosis. Changes in plasma proteins – presence of a paraprotein (as in myeloma) – may cause a rise in MCV without macrocytes being present in the blood film. Drugs that affect DNA synthesis – for example, hydroxycarbamide (hydroxyurea) and azathioprine – can cause macrocytosis with or without megaloblastic changes. Indeed, failure of the MCV to be raised in a patient prescribed hydroxycarbamide suggests lack of compliance with the drug. Finally, a rare, benign familial type of macrocytosis has been described.

Box 2.3 **Other causes of macrocytosis.**

The following are usually associated with a normoblastic marrow:
- Alcohol
- Myelodysplasia
- Liver disease
- Cytotoxic drugs
- Hypothyroidism
- Paraproteinaemia (such as myeloma)
- Reticulocytosis
- Pregnancy
- Aplastic anaemia
- Neonatal period
- Red cell aplasia

Diagnosis

Patients with macrocytosis may need to undergo a number of investigations (Box 2.4).

Biochemical assays

The most widely used screening tests for the deficiencies are the serum B_{12} and folate assays. A low serum concentration implies deficiency, but a subnormal serum concentration may occur in the absence of pronounced body deficiency – for example, in pregnancy (vitamin B_{12}) and with recent poor dietary intake (folate).

Red cell folate can also be used to screen for folate deficiency; a low concentration usually implies appreciable depletion of body folate, but the concentration also falls in severe B_{12} deficiency, so it is more difficult to interpret the significance of a low red cell than serum folate concentration in patients with megaloblastic anaemia. Moreover, if the patient has received a recent blood transfusion the red cell folate concentration will partly reflect the folate concentration of the transfused red cells.

Specialist investigations

Assays of serum homocysteine (raised in B_{12} or folate deficiency) or methylmalonic acid (raised in B_{12} deficiency) are used in some specialised laboratories. Serum homocysteine levels are also raised in renal failure and with certain drugs (e.g. corticosteroids), and they increase with age and smoking. The normal ranges in different age groups are not well established for these tests and are generally not used in routine diagnosis.

Autoantibodies

For patients with B_{12} or folate deficiency it is important to establish the underlying cause. In PA, intrinsic factor antibodies are present in plasma in 50% of patients and parietal cell antibodies in 90% of patients. Parietal cell antibody is also positive in patients with autoimmune gastritis without PA, but intrinsic factor antibodies are specific for PA. Serum gastrin levels are substantially raised in PA and usually less markedly in milder forms of autoimmune gastritis. Anti-endomysial and anti-transglutaminase antibodies are usually positive in gluten-induced enteropathy.

Box 2.4 **Laboratory investigations that may be needed in patients with macrocytosis.**

- Serum vitamin B_{12} assay
- Serum (and red cell) folate assay
- Liver and thyroid function
- Reticulocyte count
- Serum protein electrophoresis
- For vitamin B_{12} deficiency: serum parietal cell and intrinsic factor antibodies, serum gastrin concentration
- For folate deficiency: anti-endomysial and anti-transglutaminase antibodies
- Consider bone marrow examination for megaloblastic changes suggestive of vitamin B_{12} or folate deficiency, or alternative diagnoses (e.g. myelodysplasia, aplastic anaemia, myeloma)
- Endoscopy – gastric biopsy (vitamin B_{12} deficiency); duodenal biopsy (folate deficiency)

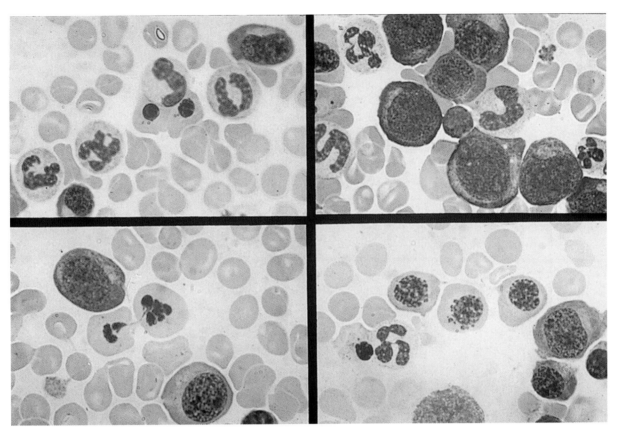

Figure 2.5 Bone marrow appearances in megaloblastic anaemia: developing red cells are larger than normal, with nuclei that are immature relative to their cytoplasm (nuclear : cytoplasmic asynchrony). Source: Reproduced with permission from *Clinical Haematology*, 3e.

Other investigations

A bone marrow examination is usually performed to confirm megaloblastic anaemia (Figure 2.5). It is also required for the diagnosis of myelodysplasia (Figure 2.6), aplastic anaemia, myeloma or with other marrow disorders associated with macrocytosis.

Endoscopy should be performed to confirm atrophic gastritis and exclude gastric carcinoma or gastric polyps, which are two to three times more common in patients with PA than in age- and sex-matched controls.

If folate deficiency is diagnosed, it is important to assess dietary folate intake and to exclude gluten-induced enteropathy by tests for serum anti-endomysial and anti-transglutaminase antibodies, endoscopy and duodenal biopsy. The deficiency is common in patients with diseases of increased cell turnover who also have a poor diet.

Treatment

Vitamin B_{12} deficiency is treated initially by giving the patient six injections of hydroxocobalamin 1 mg at intervals of about 3–4 days, followed by such injections every 3 months for life. A few advocate oral B_{12} therapy, but large doses (e.g. 1 mg cyanocobalamin daily) are needed to get a few milligrams absorbed because of the failure of physiological absorption of B_{12}; lack of lifelong compliance may also be a problem. For patients undergoing total gastrectomy or ileal resection it is sensible to start the maintenance injections from the time of operation without waiting 2–3 years for the deficiency to cause clinical problems.

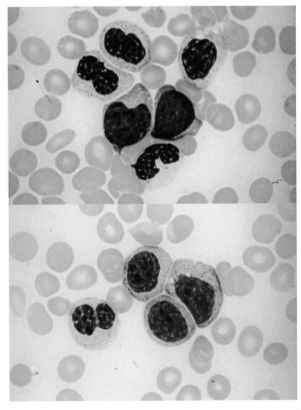

Figure 2.6 Bone marrow aspirate in myelodysplasia showing characteristic dysplastic neutrophils with bilobed nuclei.

For vegans, less frequent injections (e.g. one or two a year) may be sufficient, and the patient should be advised to eat foods to which B_{12} has been added, such as certain fortified breads or other foods.

Folate deficiency is treated with folic acid, usually 5 mg daily orally for 4 months, which is continued only if the underlying cause cannot be corrected. As prophylaxis against folate deficiency in patients with a severe haemolytic anaemia (such as sickle cell anaemia), 5 mg folic acid once weekly is probably sufficient. Vitamin B_{12} deficiency must be excluded in all patients starting folic acid treatment at these doses as such treatment may correct the anaemia in B_{12} deficiency but allow neurological disease to develop.

Further reading

Carmel R (2012) Subclinical cobalamin deficiency. *Current Opinion in Gastroenterology*, **28**, 151–158.

Devalia V, Hamilton MS and Molloy AM (2014) Guidelines for the diagnosis and treatment of cobalamin and folate disorders. *British Journal of Haematology*, **166**, 496–513.

Lachner C, Steinle NI and Regenold WT (2012) The neuropsychiatry of vitamin B_{12} deficiency in elderly patients. *Journal of Neuropsychiatry and Clinical Neuroscience*, **24**, 5–15.

Shipton MJ and Thachil J (2015) Vitamin B_{12} deficiency – a 21st century perspective. *Clinical Medicine*, **15**, 145–150.

CHAPTER 3

The Hereditary Anaemias

David J. Weatherall

MRC Weatherall Institute of Molecular Medicine, University of Oxford, Headington, Oxford, UK

OVERVIEW

- Approximately 300 000–400 000 babies with a serious inherited disorder of haemoglobin, either sickle cell anaemia or its variants or one or other form of thalassaemia, are born each year.

- Although haemoglobin disorders occur at their highest frequency in tropical countries they are encountered in most countries due to population movement from these regions.

- Neonatal screening and appropriate prophylaxis against infection can result in a significant decrease in mortality from sickle cell disease in early life.

- Carrier detection, counselling and prenatal diagnosis have reduced the number of births of children with severe β thalassaemia in many countries, and the administration of regular blood transfusions together with iron chelating agents has greatly improved the prognosis for this disease.

- The severe forms of α thalassaemia are restricted to the Far East and certain Mediterranean populations.

- The homozygous state for the severe forms of α thalassaemia results in stillbirth and a high frequency of obstetric complications.

Hereditary anaemias include disorders of the structure or synthesis of haemoglobin (Hb), deficiencies of enzymes that provide the red cell with energy or protect it from chemical damage, and abnormalities of the proteins of the red cell's membrane. Inherited diseases of Hb (haemoglobinopathies) are by far the most important.

The structure of human Hb changes during development (Figure 3.1). By the 12th week of gestation, embryonic Hb is replaced by fetal Hb (Hb F), which is slowly replaced after birth by the adult Hbs: Hb A and Hb A_2. Each type of Hb consists of two different pairs of peptide chains: Hb A has the structure $\alpha_2\beta_2$ (namely, two α chains plus two β chains), Hb A_2 has the structure $\alpha_2\delta_2$, and Hb F has the structure $\alpha_2\gamma_2$.

The haemoglobinopathies consist of structural Hb variants (the most important of which are the sickling disorders) and thalassaemias (hereditary defects of the synthesis of either the α or β globin chains).

The sickling disorders

Classification and inheritance

The common sickling disorders consist of the homozygous state for the sickle cell gene (i.e. sickle cell anaemia, Hb SS), and the compound heterozygous state for the sickle cell gene and for either Hb C (another β-chain variant) or β thalassaemia (termed Hb SC disease or sickle cell β thalassaemia) (Box 3.1). The sickle cell mutation results in a single amino acid substitution in the β globin chain; heterozygotes have one normal (βA) and one affected (βS) β chain gene and produce about 60% Hb A and 40% Hb S; homozygotes produce mainly Hb S with small amounts of Hb F. Compound heterozygotes for Hb S and Hb C produce almost equal amounts of each variant, whereas those who inherit the sickle cell gene from one parent and β thalassaemia from the other make predominantly sickle Hb (Figure 3.2).

Pathophysiology

The amino acid substitution in the β globin chain causes red cell sickling during deoxygenation, leading to increased rigidity and aggregation in the microcirculation. These changes are reflected by a haemolytic anaemia and episodes of tissue infarction (Figure 3.3).

Geographical distribution

The sickle cell gene is spread widely throughout Africa and in countries with African immigrant populations, in some Mediterranean countries, in the Middle East and in parts of India. Screening should not be restricted to people of African origin.

Clinical features

Sickle cell carriers are not anaemic and have no clinical abnormalities (Box 3.2). Patients with sickle cell anaemia have a haemolytic anaemia, with a low Hb concentration and a high reticulocyte count; the blood film shows polychromasia and sickled erythrocytes (Figure 3.3, Box 3.3). Patients adapt well to their anaemia, and it is the vascular occlusive or sequestration episodes ('crises') that pose the main threat (Box 3.4). Crises take several forms. The commonest, called the painful crisis, is associated with widespread bone

---

ABC of Clinical Haematology, Fourth Edition. Edited by Drew Provan.
© 2018 John Wiley & Sons Ltd. Published 2018 by John Wiley & Sons Ltd.

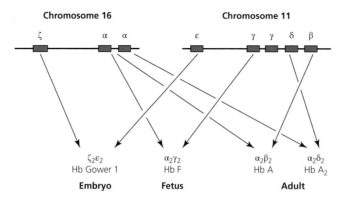

Figure 3.1 Simplified representation of the genetic control of human Hb. Because α chains are shared by both fetal and adult Hb, mutations of the α globin genes affect Hb production in both fetal and adult life; diseases that are due to defective β globin production are only manifest after birth when Hb A replaces Hb F.

Box 3.1 **Sickling syndromes.**

- Hb SS (sickle cell anaemia)
- Hb SC disease
- Hb S/β+ thalassaemia
- Hb S/β⁰ thalassaemia
- Hb SD disease

Box 3.2 **Sickle cell trait (Hb A and Hb S).**

- Less than half the Hb in each red cell is Hb S
- Occasional renal papillary necrosis
- Inability to concentrate the urine (older individuals)
- Red cells do not sickle unless oxygen saturation is <40% (rarely reached in venous blood)
- Painful crises and splenic infarction have been reported in severe hypoxia, such as in unpressurised aircraft, or under anaesthesia
- Sickling is more severe where Hb S is present with another β globin chain abnormality, such as Hb S and Hb C (Hb SC) or Hb S and Hb D (Hb SD)

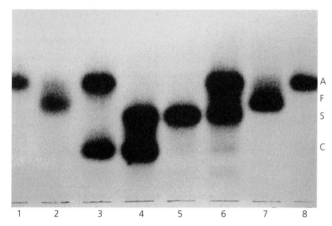

Figure 3.2 Hb electrophoresis showing (1) normal, (2) newborn, (3) Hb C trait (A–C), (4) Hb SC disease (SC), (5) sickle cell disease (SS), (6) sickle cell trait (A–S), (7) newborn, (8) normal.

Box 3.3 **Sickle cell anaemia (homozygous Hb S).**

- Anaemia (Hb 6.0–10.0 g/dL): symptoms milder than expected as Hb S has reduced oxygen affinity (i.e. gives up oxygen to tissues more easily)
- Sickled cells may be present in blood film: sickling occurs at oxygen tensions found in venous blood; cyclical sickling episodes
- Reticulocytes: raised to 10–20%
- Red cells contain ≥80% Hb S (rest is Hb F)
- Variable haemolysis
- Hand and foot syndrome (dactylitis)
- Intermittent episodes, or crises, characterised by bone pain, worsening anaemia, or pulmonary or neurological disease
- Chronic leg ulcers
- Gallstones

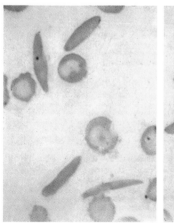 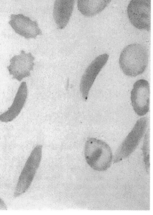

Figure 3.3 Peripheral blood film from patient with sickle cell anaemia showing sickled erythrocytes.

pain and is usually self-limiting. More serious and life-threatening crises include the sequestration of red cells into the lung or spleen, strokes, or red cell aplasia associated with parvovirus infections.

Diagnosis

Sickle cell anaemia should be suspected in any patient of an appropriate racial group with a haemolytic anaemia. It can be confirmed by a sickle cell test, although this does not distinguish between heterozygotes and homozygotes. A definitive diagnosis requires Hb electrophoresis and the demonstration of the sickle cell trait in both parents.

Prevention and treatment

Pregnant women in at-risk racial groups should be screened in early pregnancy; if the woman and her partner are carriers they should be offered either prenatal or neonatal diagnosis. As soon as the diagnosis is established, babies should receive penicillin daily and be immunised against *Streptococcus pneumoniae*, *Haemophilus influenzae* type b and *Neisseria meningitidis*. Parents should be warned to seek medical advice on any suspicion of infection. Painful crises should be managed with adequate analgesics, hydration and oxygen. The patient should be observed carefully for a source of infection and a drop in Hb concentration. Pulmonary sequestration crises require urgent exchange transfusion together with oxygen therapy. Strokes should be treated with an exchange transfusion; there is now good evidence that they can be prevented by regular surveillance of cerebral blood flow by Doppler examination and prophylactic transfusion. There is also good evidence that the frequency of painful crises can be reduced by maintaining patients on hydroxyurea, although, because of the uncertainty about the long-term effects of this form of therapy, it should be restricted to adults or, if it is used in children, should be used only for a short period. Aplastic crises require urgent blood transfusion. Splenic sequestration crises require transfusion and, because they may recur, splenectomy is advised (Box 3.5).

Sickling variants

Hb SC disease is characterised by a mild anaemia and fewer crises. Important microvascular complications, however, include retinal damage and blindness, aseptic necrosis of the femoral heads and recurrent haematuria. The disease is occasionally complicated by pulmonary embolic disease, particularly during and after pregnancy; these episodes should be treated by immediate exchange transfusion. Patients with Hb SC should have annual ophthalmological surveillance; the retinal vessel proliferation can be controlled with laser treatment. The management of the symptomatic forms of sickle cell β thalassaemia is similar to that of sickle cell anaemia.

The thalassaemias

Classification

The thalassaemias are classified as α or β thalassaemias, depending on which pair of globin chains is synthesised inefficiently. Rarer forms affect both β and δ chain production: δβ thalassaemias.

Distribution

The disease is broadly distributed throughout parts of Africa, the Mediterranean region, the Middle East, the Indian subcontinent and South East Asia, and it occurs sporadically in all racial groups (Figure 3.4). Like sickle cell anaemia, it is thought to be common because the mutation protects carriers against malaria.

Inheritance

The β thalassaemias result from over 200 different mutations of the β globin genes, which reduce the output of β globin chains, either completely (β^0 thalassaemia) or partially (β^+ thalassaemia). They are inherited in the same way as sickle cell anaemia; carrier parents have a one-in-four chance of having a homozygous child. The genetics of the α thalassaemias is more complicated because normal people have two α globin genes on each of their chromosomes 16. If both are lost (α^0 thalassaemia) no α globin chains are made, whereas if only one of the pair is lost (α^+ thalassaemia) the output of α globin chains is reduced (Figure 3.5). Impaired α globin production leads to excess γ or β chains that form unstable and physiologically useless tetramers: γ_4 (Hb Bart's) and β_4 (Hb H) (Figure 3.6). The homozygous state for α^0 thalassaemia results in the Hb Bart's hydrops syndrome, whereas the inheritance of α^0 and α^+ thalassaemia produces Hb H disease.

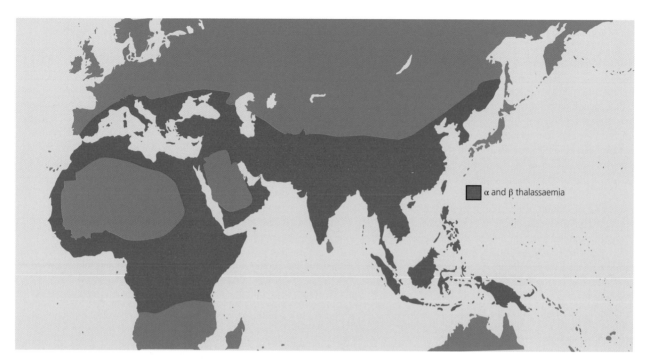

Figure 3.4 Distribution of the thalassaemias (red area).

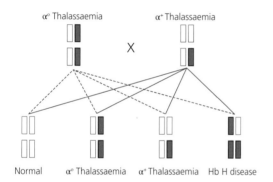

Figure 3.5 Inheritance of Hb disease (open boxes represent normal α globin genes and red boxes deleted α globin genes).

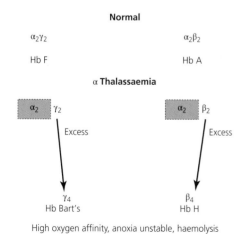

Figure 3.6 Pathophysiology of α thalassaemia.

The β thalassaemias

Heterozygotes for β thalassaemia are asymptomatic, have hypochromic microcytic red cells with a low mean cell Hb and mean cell volume (Figure 3.7), and have a mean Hb A_2 level of about twice that of normal (Box 3.6). Homozygotes, or those who have inherited a different β thalassaemia gene from both parents, usually develop severe anaemia in the first year of life (Box 3.7). This results from a deficiency of β globin chains; excess α chains precipitate in the red cell precursors, leading to their damage, either in the bone marrow or the peripheral blood. Hypertrophy of the ineffective bone marrow leads to skeletal changes, and there is variable hepatosplenomegaly. The Hb F level is always raised. If these children are transfused, the marrow is 'switched off', and growth and development may be normal. However, they accumulate iron and may die

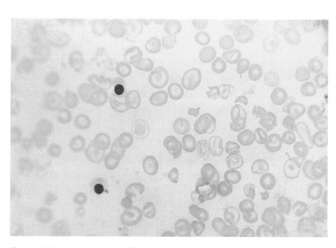

Figure 3.7 Peripheral blood film in homozygous β thalassaemia showing pronounced hypochromia and anisocytosis with nucleated red blood cells.

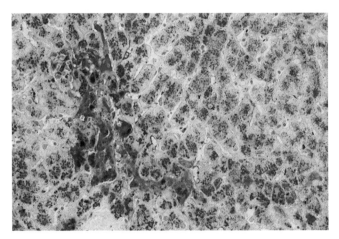

Figure 3.8 Liver biopsy from patient with β thalassaemia showing pronounced iron accumulation.

later from damage to the myocardium, pancreas or liver (Figure 3.8). They are also prone to infection and folic acid deficiency.

Milder forms of β thalassaemia (thalassaemia intermedia), although not transfusion dependent, are often associated with similar bone changes, anaemia, leg ulcers and delayed development. The most important form of β thalassaemia intermedia is Hb E β thalassaemia, which results from the inheritance of Hb E and a β thalassaemia gene. This condition is the commonest form of severe thalassaemia in many parts of Asia and is associated with a remarkably diverse clinical course; some patients are transfusion dependent, while others may remain asymptomatic.

The α thalassaemias

The Hb Bart's hydrops fetalis syndrome is characterised by the stillbirth of a severely oedematous (hydropic) fetus in the second half of pregnancy. Hb H disease is associated with a moderately severe haemolytic anaemia. The carrier states for α^0 thalassaemia and the homozygous state for α$^+$ thalassaemia result in a mild hypochromic anaemia with normal Hb A$_2$ levels (Box 3.8). They can only be distinguished with certainty by DNA analysis in a specialised laboratory. In addition to the aforementioned distribution, α thalassaemia is also seen in European populations in association with mental retardation; the molecular pathology is quite different to the common inherited forms of the condition. There are two major forms of α thalassaemia associated with mental retardation (ATR): one encoded on chromosome 16 (ATR-16) and the other on the X chromosome (ATR-X). ATR-16 is usually associated with mild mental retardation and is due to loss of the α globin genes together with other genetic material from the end of the short arm of chromosome 16. ATR-X is associated with more severe mental retardation and a variety of skeletal deformities, and is encoded by a gene on the X chromosome, which is expressed widely in different tissues during different stages of development. These conditions should be suspected in any infant or child with retarded development who has the haematological picture of a mild α thalassaemia trait.

Prevention and treatment

As β thalassaemia is easily identified in heterozygotes, pregnant women of appropriate racial groups should be screened; if a woman is found to be a carrier, her partner should be tested and the couple counselled. Prenatal diagnosis by chorionic villus sampling can be carried out between the ninth and 13th weeks of pregnancy (Box 3.9). Babies with β thalassaemia major should be observed very carefully regarding growth, activity and steady-state Hb level.

When it is certain that they require regular transfusion, they should be given washed red cell transfusions at monthly intervals; it is vital that the blood is screened for human immunodeficiency virus/acquired immunodeficiency syndrome, hepatitis B and C viruses and, in some countries, malaria.

To prevent iron overload, overnight infusions of desferrioxamine together with vitamin C should be started, and the patient's serum ferritin, or better, hepatic iron concentrations, should be monitored; complications of desferrioxamine include infections with *Yersinia* spp., retinal and acoustic nerve damage and reduction in growth associated with calcification of the vertebral discs.

The recently developed oral chelating agent deferasirox has been subjected to a number of clinical trials that suggest its efficacy in maintaining reduced hepatic iron concentration is comparable to that of desferrioxamine. Its very long-term effect on the control of iron accumulation remains to be determined. Because of potential renal or other complications it is advised that patients who receive this drug should have serum creatinine, amino transferases and bilirubin levels assessed monthly. The other oral chelating agent, deferiprone, is not so effective at maintaining safe hepatic iron levels and is associated with complications, including agranulocytosis, arthritis and neurological abnormalities. Although it has been reported to be of particular value in unloading cardiac iron, the American Food and Drug Administration has recently reported that there are no controlled trials demonstrating a direct treatment benefit. In patients who receive deferiprone it is advised that they undergo weekly assessment of complete blood counts and monthly assessment of serum amino transferases. Bone marrow transplantation, if appropriate HLA-DR-matched siblings are available, may carry a good prognosis if carried out early in life. Treatment with agents designed to raise the production of Hb F is still at the experimental stage.

In β thalassaemia and Hb H disease, progressive splenomegaly or increasing blood requirements, or both, indicate that splenectomy may be beneficial. Patients who undergo splenectomy should be vaccinated against *S. pneumoniae*, *H. influenzae* and *N. meningitidis* preoperatively, and should receive a maintenance dose of oral penicillin indefinitely.

Red cell enzyme defects

Red cells have two main metabolic pathways, one burning glucose anaerobically to produce energy, the other generating reduced glutathione to protect against injurious oxidants. Many inherited enzyme defects have been described. Some of those of the energy pathway (e.g. pyruvate kinase deficiency) cause haemolytic anaemia; any child with this type of anaemia from birth should be referred to a centre capable of analysing the major red cell enzymes. Glucose-6-phosphate dehydrogenase (G6PD) deficiency involves the protective pathway. It affects millions of people worldwide, mainly the same racial groups as are affected by the thalassaemias. G6PD deficiency is sex linked and affects predominantly males (Box 3.10). It causes neonatal jaundice, sensitivity to broad (fava) beans and haemolytic responses to oxidant drugs.

Red cell membrane defects

The red cell membrane is a complex sandwich of proteins that are required to maintain the integrity of the cell. There are many inherited defects of the membrane proteins, some of which cause haemolytic anaemia. Hereditary spherocytosis is due to a structural change that makes the cells leakier. It is particularly important to identify this disease because it can be 'cured' by splenectomy. There are many rare inherited varieties of elliptical or oval red cells, some associated with chronic haemolysis and response to splenectomy. A child with chronic haemolytic anaemia with abnormally shaped red cells should always be referred for expert advice.

Box 3.9 **Women with thalassaemia.**

- Women with the haematological features of thalassaemia trait with normal Hb A$_2$ levels should be referred to a centre able to identify the different forms of α thalassaemia
- Those with α^0 thalassaemia trait, if their partners are similarly affected, should be referred for prenatal diagnosis
- This is because the Hb Bart's hydrops syndrome is associated with an increased risk of toxaemia of pregnancy and post-partum bleeding due to a hypertrophied placenta

---

Box 3.10 **Drugs causing haemolysis in patients with G6PD deficiency.**

Antimalarials
- Primiquine
- Pamaquine

Analgesics*
- Phenacetin
- Acetylsalicylic acid

Others
- Sulphonamides
- Nalidixic acid
- Dapsone

* Probably only at high doses.

Other hereditary anaemias

Other anaemias with an important inherited component include Fanconi's anaemia (hypoplastic anaemia with skeletal deformities), Blackfan–Diamond anaemia (red cell aplasia) and several forms of congenital dyserythropoietic anaemia.

Further reading

Luzzatto L and Karadimitris A (2010) The molecular basis of anemia. In *Molecular Hematology*, 3rd edn (ed. D Provan and JG Gribben), Wiley-Blackwell, Oxford, pp. 140–164.

Luzzatto L and Poggi V (2009) Glucose-6-phosphate dehydrogenase deficiency. In *Hematology of Infancy and Childhood*, 7th edn (ed. SH Orkin, DG Nathan, D Ginsburg *et al.*), Saunders Elsevier, Philadelphia, PA, pp. 883–910.

Steinberg MH, Forget BG, Higgs DR and Weatherall DJ (2009) *Disorders of Haemoglobin*, 2nd edn, Cambridge University Press, New York.

Weatherall DJ and Clegg JB (2001) *The Thalassemia Syndromes*, 4th edn, Blackwell Publishing, Oxford.

Weatherall DJ, Schechter AN and Nathan DJ (2013) *Hemoglobin and Its Diseases*. Cold Spring Harbor Laboratory Press.

CHAPTER 4

Polycythaemia Vera, Essential Thrombocythaemia and Myelofibrosis

Anna L. Godfrey[1], George S. Vassiliou[2,3] and Anthony R. Green[3,4]

[1] Department of Haematology, Cambridge University Hospitals NHS Foundation Trust, Cambridge, UK
[2] Wellcome Trust Sanger Institute, Wellcome Genome Campus, Hinxton, Cambridge, UK
[3] Wellcome Trust/MRC Cambridge Stem Cell Institute, University of Cambridge, Cambridge, UK
[4] Department of Haematology, University of Cambridge, Cambridge, UK

OVERVIEW

- The myeloproliferative neoplasms (MPNs) comprise polycythaemia vera (PV), essential thrombocythaemia (ET) and primary myelofibrosis (PMF).

- They are closely related clonal blood disorders of haemopoietic stem cells.

- Appropriately treated PV and ET are compatible with long-term survival, whereas life expectancy is significantly reduced in PMF.

- Arterial and venous thromboses are the commonest cause of morbidity and mortality in the MPNs.

- A mutation in the tyrosine kinase JAK2 (*JAK2 V617F*) is found in many patients with MPNs, including almost all with PV, whilst mutations in *CALR* and *MPL* account for smaller proportions of patients with ET and PMF.

- Patients with PV and ET are treated with low-dose aspirin and risk stratified according to their risk of thrombosis, with those at high risk being treated with additional cytoreductive drugs such as hydroxycarbamide.

- In PV the haematocrit should be maintained below 0.45; venesection is used in many patients and may be sufficient, without cytoreduction, in patients at low risk of vascular events.

- Treatments for PMF include JAK inhibitors, allogeneic stem cell transplantation and supportive care, including blood transfusion.

- The MPNs have an inherent risk of progression to acute leukaemia, which is most significant in PMF.

Polycythaemia vera (PV), essential thrombocythaemia (ET) and primary myelofibrosis (PMF), known collectively as the classical myeloproliferative neoplasms (MPNs), are clonal disorders originating from a neoplastic haematopoietic stem cell. They are most common in middle or older age and share several features, including a potential to transform into acute myeloid leukaemia and into each other. Treatment of PV and ET can greatly influence prognosis, hence the importance of differentiating them from non-clonal conditions associated with raised haemoglobin (erythrocytosis) or a raised platelet count (thrombocytosis), whose prognosis and treatment are different. Myelofibrosis may arise *de novo* (PMF) or result from progression of PV or ET.

Molecular pathogenesis of myeloproliferative neoplasms

In 2005, acquired activating mutations in the gene for the tyrosine kinase JAK2, leading to a valine to phenylalanine substitution at amino acid 617 (V617F), were identified in nearly all cases of PV and approximately half of patients with ET or PMF. The abnormally active mutant JAK2 is thought to amplify signalling downstream of cytokine receptors and thus have a central role in the pathogenesis of MPNs. Most patients with PV who lack the *JAK2 V617F* mutation were later found to carry alternative mutations, within exon 12 of *JAK2*, which may have similar biochemical consequences. Additional mutations were subsequently discovered in the *MPL* gene in approximately 5–10% of patients with ET or PMF. This gene encodes the thrombopoietin receptor, and these mutations again appear to activate this signalling pathway. Most recently, mutations in the gene for calreticulin, *CALR*, have been reported in approximately 25–35% of patients with ET and PMF. Calreticulin is a multifunctional protein that normally resides within the endoplasmic reticulum. The mechanism by which these mutations, all of which generate a novel C-terminal peptide sequence, cause MPNs is not yet fully established.

Testing for mutations in these genes has become an established part of the diagnosis of PV, ET and PMF and of distinguishing these conditions from reactive or non-clonal causes of abnormal blood counts.

ABC of Clinical Haematology, Fourth Edition. Edited by Drew Provan.
© 2018 John Wiley & Sons Ltd. Published 2018 by John Wiley & Sons Ltd.

Erythrocytosis and polycythaemia vera

An elevation in haematocrit defines erythrocytosis (Figure 4.1). A raised haematocrit (>0.52 in men, >0.48 in women) needs to be confirmed on a specimen taken without prolonged venous stasis (tourniquet), and patients with a persistently raised haematocrit require further assessment. This begins with history and examination to identify factors that may cause a secondary erythrocytosis (Box 4.1). In the absence of a clear secondary cause (e.g. severe hypoxic lung disease), an early key investigation comprises mutation screening of the *JAK2* gene (Figure 4.2). The finding of a *JAK2* mutation in the presence of a raised haematocrit is sufficient to confirm the diagnosis of PV.

In patients negative for *JAK2* mutations, further investigations should seek to exclude an *apparent erythrocytosis*. This condition is characterised by a raised haematocrit but without an increased red cell mass and is caused by a reduction in plasma volume. Red cell mass is best expressed as the percentage difference between the measured value and that predicted for the patient's height and weight (derived from tables). Red cell mass measurements greater than 25% above the predicted value constitute *true erythrocytosis*. In patients with a moderately raised haematocrit, a red cell mass estimation can be very helpful in determining whether a true erythrocytosis is in fact present. However in those with a very high haematocrit (>0.60 in men or >0.56 in women), this invariably predicts a raised red cell mass and formal estimation is unnecessary.

In patients with a true erythrocytosis who are negative for *JAK2* mutations, additional investigations (Figure 4.2) should seek to identify a possible secondary or familial cause (Box 4.1).

Polycythaemia vera

Presentation

This can be incidental, but is classically associated with a history of occlusive vascular lesions (stroke, transient ischaemic attack, ischaemic digits, venous thrombosis), headache, mental clouding, facial redness, itching, abnormal bleeding or gout. Palpable splenomegaly may be detected on clinical examination.

Investigations

A raised white cell count (>10 × 10⁹/L neutrophils) or a raised platelet count (>400 × 10⁹/L) suggests primary polycythaemia, especially if both are raised in the absence of an obvious cause, such as infection or carcinoma. Serum ferritin concentration should be determined as iron deficiency may mask a raised haematocrit.

Patients should be tested for *JAK2* mutations as an early step, since the identification of a mutation in the presence of a raised haematocrit (>0.52 in men, >0.48 in women) is sufficient to confirm the diagnosis of PV. Serum erythropoietin levels are typically suppressed and many patients will also undergo a bone marrow biopsy to confirm the presence of characteristic histological features.

Treatment

Patients should receive low-dose aspirin, which has been shown to reduce the risk of thrombotic events in PV (Box 4.2). Other cardiovascular risk factors, such as hypertension, diabetes mellitus and hypercholesterolaemia, should be managed intensively and

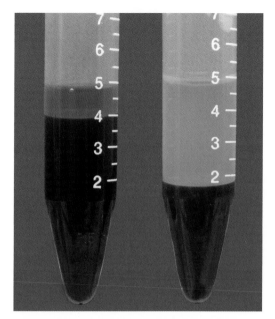

Figure 4.1 Raised PCV in a patient with PV (left) compared with a blood sample from a person with a normal PCV (right).

Box 4.1 **Causes of true erythrocytosis.**

Familial/inherited
- High oxygen-affinity haemoglobin
- 2,3-Bisphosphoglycerate mutase deficiency
- Mutations in the oxygen sensing pathway, e.g. *VHL, PHD2, HIF-2α* genes
- Activating mutations in the erythropoietin receptor gene, *EPOR*

Acquired

Primary
- PV

Secondary
- Chronic tissue hypoxia
  - Lung disease
  - Obstructive sleep apnoea
  - Congenital cyanotic heart disease
  - Abnormal oxygen transport (e.g. carboxyhaemoglobinaemia in heavy smokers)
- Local renal hypoxia (e.g. renal cysts, hydronephrosis, renal artery stenosis)
- Ectopic erythropoietin production
  - Renal tumours
  - Extrarenal neoplasms (e.g. cerebellar haemangioblastoma, hepatoma)
- Endocrine causes
  - Exogenous hormones (e.g. androgenic steroids, erythropoietin)
  - Endogenous syndromes (e.g. Cushing's and Conn's syndromes – rarely)

patients should be advised not to smoke. Therapy to maintain the haematocrit at <0.45 has also been shown to reduce the risk of vascular events. Haematocrit control may be achieved through

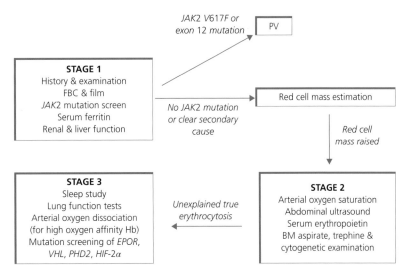

Figure 4.2 Algorithm for investigation of a patient presenting with a raised haematocrit. Note that red cell mass estimation is unnecessary if the haematocrit is >0.6 in men or >0.56 in women. Source: Adapted from McMullin MF, Reilly JT, Campbell P *et al.* (2007) Amendment to the guideline for diagnosis and investigation of polycythaemia/erythrocytosis. *British Journal of Haematology*, **138**, 821–822.

Box 4.2 Principles of management in PV and ET.

- Management of cardiovascular risk factors
- Low-dose aspirin unless contraindicated (caution if platelet count >1000 × 10^9/L)
- Haematocrit control to <0.45 in PV
- Cytoreduction in patients at high risk of vascular events:
  - Age >60 years
  - Previous history of thrombosis
  - Platelet count >1500 × 10^9/L
  - Additional indications for each disease are noted in the text

---

venesection, which is often required frequently at first, but eventually only every 6–10 weeks in most patients. Additional treatment with cytoreductive therapy is recommended for patients at high risk of vascular events (Box 4.2), as well as for those with marked thrombocytosis, symptomatic splenomegaly, constitutional symptoms or progressive leucocytosis. Hydroxycarbamide (0.5–2 g daily) is recommended for this purpose as it is usually well tolerated and is not thought to have a pronounced leukaemogenic potential. Interferon-α is an alternative in younger patients and may be preferred as it is theoretically even less likely to carry a leukaemogenic risk. Anagrelide can specifically reduce the platelet count but should be used with caution (see 'Essential thrombocythaemia' section). Treatment with radioactive phosphorus (^{32}P) has been superseded because of the additional risk of inducing malignancies, including acute leukaemia, in later life, although oral busulphan may be a convenient drug in elderly patients.

Prognosis

Adequately treated patients with PV have a long median survival (>10 years), but there is also a 20% incidence of transformation to myelofibrosis and 5–10% to acute leukaemia. The incidence of leukaemia is further increased in those who have transformed to myelofibrosis and those treated with ^{32}P or multiple cytotoxic agents.

Secondary erythrocytosis

Many causes of secondary erythrocytosis have been identified. The commonest are chronic hypoxia and renal diseases, the kidneys being the site of erythropoietin production (Box 4.1). The abuse of drugs such as erythropoietin and anabolic steroids may need to be considered in the correct context. These conditions are associated with a raised serum erythropoietin level, or one which is inappropriately normal in the presence of erythrocytosis. Investigations aim to determine the underlying disorder to which the erythrocytosis is secondary.

Treatment

This is aimed at removing the underlying cause when practicable. In most cases of secondary erythrocytosis the risk of vascular occlusion is much less pronounced than in PV, and venesection is usually undertaken only in those with a very high haematocrit. In practice, the symptoms experienced by individual patients often dictate the target haematocrit. In erythrocytosis associated with renal lesions or other tumours, the haematocrit should generally be reduced to <0.45.

Apparent erythrocytosis

In apparent or relative erythrocytosis, red cell mass is not increased and the raised haematocrit is secondary to a decrease in plasma volume. An association exists with smoking, alcohol excess, obesity, diuretics and hypertension.

The need for treatment is uncertain. On follow-up, up to one-third of patients spontaneously revert to a normal haematocrit.

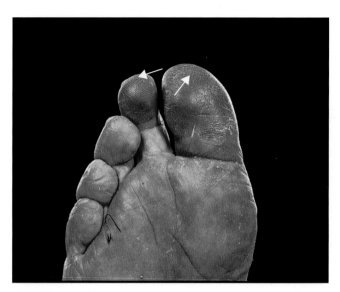

Figure 4.3 Toe ischaemia in a patient with ET.

Thrombocytosis

A raised platelet count (thrombocytosis) most commonly represents a reactive response to one or more of a diverse group of stimuli, such as iron deficiency, inflammation, infection or recent surgery. Additionally, thrombocytosis can be due to one of several clonal blood disorders (Box 4.3).

Essential thrombocythaemia

A persistent platelet count above 450×10^9/L is the central diagnostic feature, but other reactive and clonal causes of a raised platelet count should be excluded before a diagnosis of ET can be made. The diagnosis should not be missed, however, as unlike reactive thrombocytosis, where the risk is small, ET carries a high risk of occlusive vascular events.

Presentation

Presentation is often incidental. Of the patients with ET, 30–50% have microvascular occlusive events such as burning pain in the extremities (erythromelalgia) or digital ischaemia, major vascular occlusive events, or haemorrhage at presentation (Figure 4.3). Palpable splenomegaly may be present but is not prominent in most patients.

Laboratory investigations

The *JAK2 V617F* mutation is found in about half the cases of this disorder, and mutations in the *CALR* and *MPL* genes in a smaller proportion. Given that a molecular abnormality can be identified in approximately 85% of cases of ET, these investigations comprise an important part of the diagnostic pathway (Figure 4.4). In such cases, if PV and PMF can be ruled out, a diagnosis of ET can be confidently made. In the absence of a molecular abnormality, investigations should aim to exclude other causes of thrombocytosis. Apart from a full blood count and blood film, these should include erythrocyte sedimentation rate, serum C-reactive protein, serum ferritin and bone marrow aspirate, trephine and cytogenetic analysis. Trephine histology can often reveal features such as clusters of large megakaryocytes that are suggestive of ET (Figure 4.5). Cytogenetic studies are generally normal in ET, but occasionally

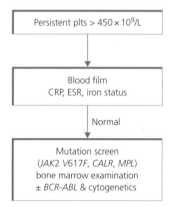

Figure 4.4 Algorithm for investigation of a patient presenting with a raised platelet count. Source: Adapted from Harrison *et al.* (2010).

Persistent plts > 450×10^9/L

↓

Blood film
CRP, ESR, iron status

↓ Normal

Mutation screen
(*JAK2 V617F*, *CALR*, *MPL*)
bone marrow examination
± *BCR-ABL* & cytogenetics

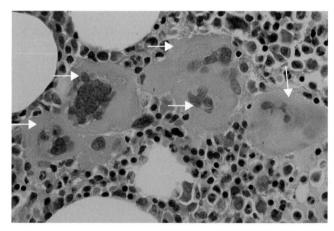

Figure 4.5 Bone marrow trephine biopsy from a patient with ET showing clustering of large megakaryocytes (arrows).

patients with chronic myeloid leukaemia will present with an isolated thrombocytosis, so a *BCR–ABL* fusion should be excluded. Certain cytogenetic abnormalities may also favour an alternative diagnosis of myelodysplasia.

Treatment and prognosis

All patients should receive daily low-dose aspirin, unless contraindicated because of allergy, bleeding or peptic ulceration. This reduces the risk of vascular occlusion, but may increase the risk of haemorrhage, and caution is required in those with a very marked thrombocytosis (platelets >1000 × 10⁹/L). Other cardiovascular risk factors should be managed aggressively.

Reduction of the platelet count with cytoreductive agents is recommended in those at high risk of vascular events (Box 4.2) as it has been shown to reduce the incidence of thrombotic complications. Cytoreduction may also be required in younger patients in the presence of symptomatic splenomegaly, erythromelalgia or microvascular symptoms that persist despite aspirin therapy. Hydroxycarbamide is typically used as a first-line treatment. Anagrelide is a platelet-specific agent, but as it appears to be less effective in reducing venous thromboses and to marginally increase the risk of transformation to myelofibrosis it should be used as a second-line treatment. Interferon-α has also been used and is particularly useful in pregnancy. Intermittent low-dose oral busulphan is an alternative treatment in the most elderly patients.

The risk of thrombotic events in ET varies from approximately 3% to 11% per year, primarily depending on the age of the patient and whether there is a history of previous thrombosis. Other factors may also play a role (e.g. patients with a *JAK2* mutation have a higher risk of thrombosis than those with a *CALR* mutation). The median survival in ET is long (>15 years) but is lower than that of the age- and sex-matched population, with transformation to myelofibrosis or acute leukaemia occurring in a minority of patients.

Primary myelofibrosis

The main features of PMF are bone marrow fibrosis, extramedullary haematopoiesis (production of blood cells in organs other than the bone marrow), splenomegaly and a leucoerythroblastic blood picture (immature red and white cells in the blood) (Figure 4.6). Good evidence exists that the fibroblast proliferation is secondary

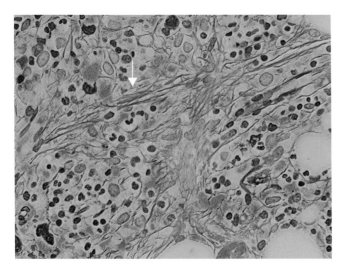

Figure 4.6 Bone marrow trephine biopsy from a patient with advanced PMF. Note the marked linear reticulin staining (e.g. arrow).

and not part of the clonal process. In some patients, the fibrosis is accompanied by new bone formation (osteomyelosclerosis). PMF needs to be distinguished from causes of secondary myelofibrosis.

Presentation

PMF can have a long pre-clinical period, and in some cases patients may have had undiagnosed PV or ET. Although the diagnosis may be made in asymptomatic patients, the absence of a palpable spleen at presentation is rare. Presenting features may include abdominal fullness or discomfort (splenomegaly), anaemia, fatigue and a bleeding diathesis. Fevers, night sweats and weight loss may be present and are associated with more advanced disease.

Laboratory investigations

Significant bone marrow fibrosis is the *sine qua non* of PMF (Figure 4.7), but this is not sufficient to make the diagnosis as additional clinical features are required (Box 4.4). A leucoerythroblastic blood picture is characteristic but not diagnostic of PMF as it can occur in cases of marrow infiltration, severe sepsis, severe haemolysis and other circumstances (Box 4.5). The blood count in PMF is

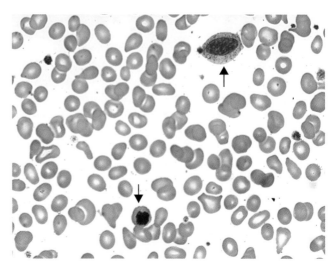

Figure 4.7 Leucoerythroblastic blood film in a patient with PMF. Note the nucleated red blood cell (lower arrow) and the myelocyte (upper arrow).

Box 4.4 **Diagnostic criteria for PMF (British Committee for Standards in Haematology, 2012).**

Diagnosis of PMF requires A1 + A2 and any two B criteria
A1. Bone marrow fibrosis ≥3 (on 0–4 scale)
A2. Pathogenetic mutation (e.g. *JAK2*, *MPL*), or absence of both *BCR–ABL1* and reactive causes of bone marrow fibrosis
B1. Palpable splenomegaly
B2. Unexplained anaemia
B3. Leucoerythroblastosis
B4. Teardrop red cells
B5. Constitutional symptoms (drenching night sweats, weight loss >10% over 6 months, unexplained fever, diffuse bone pains)
B6. Histological evidence of extramedullary haematopoiesis

variable: in the initial 'proliferative phase' red cell production may be normal or even increased, and about half of presenting patients may have a raised white cell or platelet count. However, as the bone marrow becomes more fibrotic, the more familiar 'cytopenic phase' supervenes. Mutations in *JAK2*, *CALR* or *MPL* occur in approximately 90% of cases with PMF and help to confirm the diagnosis.

Treatment and prognosis

The median survival is 5–6 years, but prognosis varies substantially between patients. A number of clinical and haematological parameters, including advanced age, anaemia and constitutional symptoms, are associated with a poorer prognosis (Box 4.6). Bone marrow transplantation from a matched sibling or unrelated donor should be offered to young patients with poor prognostic features. This is the only curative treatment modality for myelofibrosis, but in view of its toxicity it cannot be performed in the majority of patients.

Supportive blood transfusion may be needed for anaemic patients. Androgenic steroids, such as danazol and oxymethalone, can improve the haemoglobin in a proportion of anaemic patients. Cytoreductive agents, such as hydroxycarbamide, can be used in the proliferative phase, particularly if the platelet count is raised. Splenectomy or splenic radiotherapy have been used in the past to reduce the pain associated with a very enlarged spleen and/or the need for transfusions. However, these procedures carry significant risks of morbidity and mortality and are now used infrequently. More recently, a more effective strategy has been the use of oral JAK inhibitors, which can provide significant improvements in splenomegaly and constitutional symptoms. These agents are not selective for mutant JAK2 and can offer benefit to patients with or without *JAK2* mutations. JAK inhibitors do not improve anaemia, do not stop or reverse the underlying fibrotic disease process and do not prevent transformation to acute leukaemia, but nonetheless are associated with an improvement in overall survival.

Death can be due to haemorrhage, infection or transformation to acute leukaemia. Portal hypertension with varices, iron overload from blood transfusion, and compression of vital structures by extramedullary haemopoietic masses may also contribute to morbidity and mortality.

Further reading

Barbui T, Barosi G, Birgegard G *et al.* (2011) Philadelphia-negative classical myeloproliferative neoplasms: critical concepts and management recommendations from European LeukemiaNet. *Journal of Clinical Oncology*, **29**(6), 761–770.

Harrison CN, Bareford D, Butt N *et al.* (2010) Guideline for investigation and management of adults and children presenting with a thrombocytosis. *British Journal of Haematology*, **149**, 352–375.

Harrison CN, Campbell PJ and Green AR (2015) Myeloproliferative neoplasms. In *Postgraduate Haematology* (eds AV Hoffbrand, DR Higgs, DM Keeling and AB Mehta), Blackwell Publishing, Oxford, chapter 26.

McMullin MF, Bareford D, Campbell P *et al.* (2005) Guidelines for the diagnosis, investigation and management of polycythaemia/erythrocytosis. *British Journal of Haematology*, **130**, 174–195.

Reilly JT, McMullin MF, Beer PA *et al.* (2012) Guideline for the diagnosis and management of myelofibrosis. *British Journal of Haematology*, **158**, 453–471.

CHAPTER 5

Chronic Myeloid Leukaemia

Jenny L. Byrne

Nottingham University Hospitals NHS Trust, Nottingham, UK

OVERVIEW

- Detection of the *BCR–ABL* fusion gene is diagnostic of chronic myeloid leukaemia (CML), and its product, the BCR–ABL oncoprotein, is an activated tyrosine kinase which causes the leukaemia.

- The *BCR–ABL* fusion gene is formed as a result of a reciprocal translocation between the long arms of chromosomes 9 and 22, known as the Philadelphia chromosome, or t(9;22)(q34;q11).

- Without treatment CML can progress from the chronic phase to blast crisis, which has a very poor prognosis.

- Tyrosine kinase inhibitors (TKIs), such as imatinib, can lead to cytogenetic remissions and deep molecular responses in a high percentage of patients.

- *BCR–ABL* mutations are the commonest cause of resistance to TKIs, and allogeneic transplantation is reserved for patients who fail to respond to TKIs.

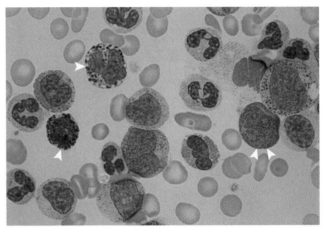

Figure 5.1 Typical blood film in chronic phase (CP) CML showing many mature granulocytes, myelocytes, basophils (arrow) and a blast cell (double arrow).

Clinical features

Chronic myeloid leukaemia (CML) is a myeloproliferative neoplasm with an incidence if 1–2 per 100 000 population, averaging 700 new cases in the UK each year. Presentation may be at any age, but it is very rare in children, and peaks between the ages of 50 and 70 years, with a slight male predominance. Approximately 30–50% of patients are asymptomatic at diagnosis and are diagnosed by routine physical examination or blood tests done for a different reason.

The disease arises from a defect in a single haemopoietic stem cell which then has a proliferative advantage over the normal stem cells, resulting in a gradual build-up of the leukaemic cells over months or years. By the time that the disease is diagnosed the bone marrow is grossly hypercellular and there is a marked leucocytosis in the peripheral blood, often with a basophilia (Figure 5.1). There is also usually an associated anaemia and thrombocytosis, which may be marked. Infiltration of the spleen results in splenomegaly in 50–60% of cases (Figure 5.2).

Three distinct phases of CML are recognised: stable chronic phase (CP), and the more advanced phases, termed accelerated phase and blast crisis (Figure 5.3). The vast majority of patients are diagnosed in CP, which may last for several years, even if untreated. Where symptoms are present at all in CP they are due to the associated anaemia and splenomegaly, and include fatigue, weight loss, sweating, early satiety and left upper quadrant fullness or pain. Rare manifestations include bleeding (due to platelet dysfunction as thrombocytopenia is unusual), thrombosis, gout, priapism (due to marked leucocytosis) and retinal haemorrhages. Despite the elevated white cell count (often exceeding 100×10^9/L) features of leucostasis are rare in CP, and infections are uncommon as the white cells function normally. Headaches, bone pain, fever and arthralgias are suggestive of CML transformation, which is characterised by increasing organ infiltration, progressive splenomegaly, cytopenias and an increasing percentage of primitive or blast cells in the blood and marrow. Most patients transit through a period of accelerated phase prior to entering the blast phase, but 20% may progress to blast crisis without warning. Blast phase is rapidly fatal without treatment.

ABC of Clinical Haematology, Fourth Edition. Edited by Drew Provan.

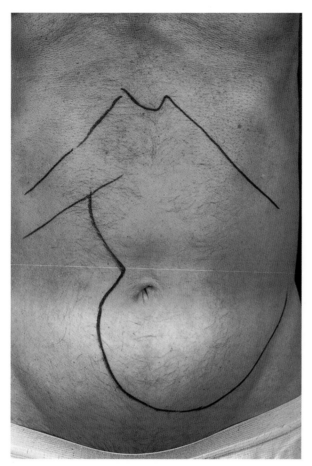

Figure 5.2 Massive splenomegaly in CP CML.

Pathophysiology

Back in 1960, cytogeneticists in Philadelphia identified a specific cytogenetic abnormality in patients with CML which they termed the Philadelphia (Ph) chromosome. Later it was discovered that the Ph chromosome was derived from a normal chromosome 22 which has lost part of its long arm as a result of a balanced reciprocal translocation between the long arm of chromosome 22 and the long arm of chromosome 9, t(9;22). Despite the additional material from chromosome 9, the resulting Ph chromosome (22q–) is shorter than its normal chromosome 22 counterpart, and the resulting chromosome 9q + is longer than the normal chromosome 9 (Figure 5.4).

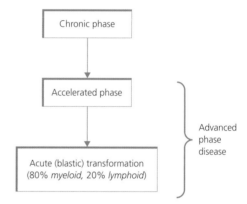

Figure 5.3 Phases of CML.

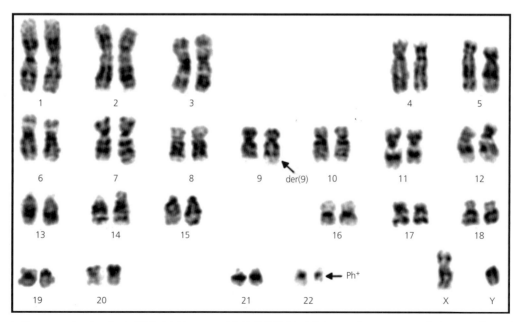

Figure 5.4 G-banded karyotype showing classical Philadelphia pattern 46,XY,t(9;22)(q34;q11). Source: *European Journal of Haematology* Volume 87, Issue 5, pages 381–393, 2 OCT 2011 DOI: 10.1111/j.1600-0609.2011.01689.x.

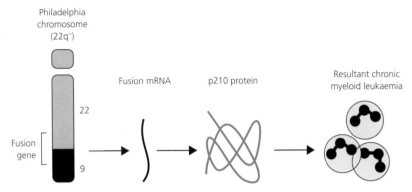

Figure 5.5 Formation of the Philadelphia chromosome resulting in a *BCR–ABL* fusion gene that generates a fusion protein (p210) responsible for the CML phenotype.

This reciprocal translocation results in the fusion of part of the *ABL* proto-oncogene on chromosome 9 with part of the *BCR* gene on chromosome 22, forming a *BCR–ABL* fusion gene. This fusion gene is transcribed and translated into the p210BCR–ABL fusion protein, which is a constitutively active tyrosine kinase that is leukaemogenic, promoting growth and replication through downstream signalling pathways and creating cytokine-independent proliferation and aberrant apoptosis (Figure 5.5).

Diagnosis

The diagnosis of CML should be considered in any patient with an unexplained leucocytosis, basophilia or thrombocytosis. Bone marrow examination is required to assess the stage of disease by virtue of the percentage of blast cells, promyelocytes, myelocytes and neutrophils and for cytogenetic evaluation to demonstrate the presence of the Ph chromosome, either by conventional G-banding or by fluorescent in-situ hybridisation studies in which there is colocalisation of probes for both *BCR* and *ABL* genes (Figure 5.6). Additional chromosomal abnormalities may be detected in 10–15% of patients and may be a sign of clonal evolution and disease acceleration. Alternatively, the diagnosis may be made by demonstrating the presence of *BCR–ABL* transcripts by molecular reverse transcription polymerase chain reaction (PCR) studies. Quantitative PCR (Q-PCR) is a highly sensitive method for detecting low levels of *BCR–ABL* transcripts and is an ideal tool for monitoring minimal residual disease in patients on treatment.

CML must be differentiated from: a leukaemoid reaction, in which the white cells may be elevated (rarely $>50 \times 10^9$/L) as a result of infection; other myeloproliferative disorders, where the white cells rarely exceed 25×10^9/L; and chronic myelomonocytic leukaemias, where the predominant increase is in the monocytoid compartment. Rare patients with leucocytosis and splenomegaly have no demonstrable Ph chromosome or *BCR–ABL* transcripts and are said to be Ph-negative CML, which has fewer treatment options and a worse prognosis.

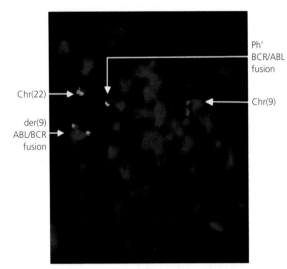

Figure 5.6 Fluorescent in-situ hybridisation showing reciprocal translocation showing *BCR–ABL* dual fusion using dual-colour probes. Source: *European Journal of Haematology* Volume 87, Issue 5, pages 381–393, 2 OCT 2011 DOI: 10.1111/j.1600-0609.2011.01689.x.

Treatment of chronic-phase disease

Initial treatment for patients with high white cell counts is usually with hydroxycarbamide, a ribonucleotide reductase inhibitor, which is effective at controlling the leucocyte count and relieving symptoms. However, it has no effect on the proportion of Ph-positive cells in the marrow and does not improve survival.

On confirming the diagnosis, the aim of therapy is to try to eradicate the Ph-positive clone. Historically, there were only two available treatments capable of achieving this goal: interferon-α, given as a subcutaneous injection several times per week, which was effective in inducing cytogenetic remissions in up to 15% of patients, but had numerous side effects; or allogeneic haemopoietic stem cell transplantation, which was limited to patients fit enough to go through the procedure and who had a suitable matched donor, and was associated with a significant morbidity and mortality.

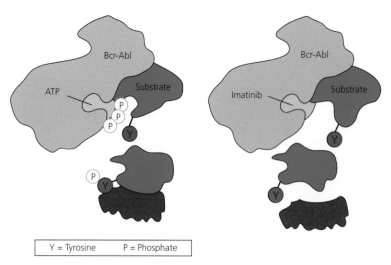

Y = Tyrosine   P = Phosphate

Figure 5.7 Mechanism of action of TKIs.

Table 5.1 Response evaluation to TKIs used as first-line therapy (European LeukaemiaNet data, 2013).

	Optimal	Warning	Failure
Baseline	—	CCA in Ph+ cells, high-risk Sokal, or Hasford score	—
3 months	Ph+ <35% and/or *BCR–ABL* <10%	Ph+ 36–95% and/or *BCR–ABL* >10%	Ph+ >95% and/or no CHR
6 months	Ph+ 0% and/or *BCR–ABL* <1%	Ph+ 1–35% and/or *BCR–ABL* 1–10%	Ph+ >35% and/or *BCR–ABL* >10%
12 months	*BCR–ABL* <0.1%	*BCR–ABL* 0.1–1%	*BCR–ABL* >1% and/or Ph+ >0%
Any time	*BCR–ABL* <0.1%	CCA in Ph– cells (–7 or 7q–)	Loss of CHR
			Loss of CCyR
			Confirmed loss of MMR
			CCA in Ph+ cells

Source: Jabbour, E. and Kantarjian, H. (2014) Chronic myeloid leukemia: 2014 update on diagnosis, monitoring, and management. *American Journal of Haematology*, **89**, 547–556. doi:10.1002/ajh.23691.
CCA: clonal chromosome abnormalities; CCyR: complete cytogenetic response; CHR: complete haematologic response; MMR: major molecular response.

The treatment of CML has advanced significantly since 1999 with the introduction of tyrosine kinase inhibitors (TKIs), such as imatinib mesylate, that block the enzymatic function of the BCR–ABL protein and kill the leukaemic cells, thus allowing regeneration of normal haemopoiesis (Figure 5.7).

Imatinib mesylate

Imatinib is given orally, at a starting dose of 400 mg once a day, and is generally well tolerated, though some patients may develop troublesome side effects, such as rash, fluid retention and gastrointestinal disturbance. Data from the pivotal IRIS study (International Randomized Study of Interferon and STI571) demonstrated the superior efficacy of imatinib over interferon combined with cytarabine. After 19 months of follow up, 76% of patients in the imatinib arm had achieved complete cytogenetic responses compared with 9% on the interferon arm ($p < 0.001$). Additionally, there was superior rate of progression-free survival (99% versus 93%, $p < 0.001$). These responses have subsequently been shown to be durable, since the 8-year follow-up data show an overall survival rate of 93% when only CML-related deaths are considered. This study led to imatinib being licensed and NICE approved for use in all phases of newly diagnosed CML.

Monitoring of patients on tyrosine kinase inhibitors

Regular monitoring using Q-PCR of *BCR–ABL* transcript numbers in the peripheral blood is required to ensure that patients are on track to achieve these responses. The European LeukaemiaNet (ELN) have published guidelines on what the 'optimal' level of molecular and cytogenetic response should be in patients being treated with TKIs at different time-points on treatment (see Table 5.1). Achievement of complete cytogenetic remission (no Ph+ metaphases detectable) and major molecular responses (Q-PCR *BCR–ABL/ABL* ratios <0.1) are desired as these are associated with a reduced risk of disease progression and superior overall survival. Additionally, recent evidence has suggested that early deep responses, defined as Q-PCR values <10% at the 3-month time-point, predict a superior outcome.

Patients who fail to achieve these responses are sub-classified into those who have sub-optimal or 'warning' levels and those who are said to have 'failed', and for whom a switch of therapy should be considered.

Second- and third-generation tyrosine kinase inhibitors

Dasatinib and nilotinib are two alternative oral second-generation TKIs that are also both licensed for use in newly diagnosed CP CML or as second-line treatments after intolerance or failure of imatinib, and both appear to be more active than imatinib. Currently, access to dasatinib in the UK is restricted to specific indications. More recently, two other TKIs, bosutinib and ponatinib, have also been licensed for patients refractory to other TKIs and show promising activity in resistant cases. Some of these newer TKIs have, however, been associated with increased side effects and toxicity, such as the development of pleural effusions with dasatinib and an increased risk of cardiovascular and peripheral vascular events with nilotinib and ponatinib. The toxicity and tolerability profiles of the different drugs need to be monitored and borne in mind when choosing drugs for individual patients.

Resistance to tyrosine kinase inhibitors

Data from the IRIS trial show that approximately 15–17% of patients treated in the CP become resistant to imatinib at some point during the course of treatment. In that study, by 8 years only 55% of patients remained on imatinib due to a combination of resistance and/or intolerance. Imatinib resistance rates are higher in more advanced phases of CML than in the CP. Although there are reported to be several mechanisms of clinical resistance to imatinib, the most common cause is the development of *BCR–ABL* kinase domain point mutations. Over 40 different *BCR–ABL* mutations have been identified, and binding of imatinib to these BCR–ABL mutants is often impaired, which leads to inadequate response or loss of response. BCR–ABL mutations are more common in secondary resistance (i.e. where patients initially appear to gain cytogenetic or molecular responses and then suddenly lose them) than in primary resistance (in which patients never appear to achieve a good cytogenetic response). Among patients with CP CML who developed secondary imatinib resistance, *BCR–ABL* mutations are reported in up to 55%.

The second-generation TKIs are able to overcome many of the mutations that confer resistance to imatinib, although there are emergent mutations which are also resistant to dasatinib and/or nilotinib. The selection of a second-line drug for a patient refractory to imatinib must take into consideration any known mutations. One mutation, the T315I mutation, or 'gate-keeper' mutation, is of particular importance since it confers resistance to all the available TKIs except ponatinib, which shows encouraging efficacy in these cases.

Allogeneic haemopoietic stem cell transplantation remains an option for patients who have failed two or more TKIs and in whom a suitable donor can be identified, although it is associated with significant morbidity and mortality. Molecular monitoring is required after transplantation to detect early relapse, which may occur in a proportion of patients. If detected early, relapse can be effectively treated with infusions of donor lymphocytes from the original donor, which may invoke 'graft versus leukaemia' responses and eradicate the relapsing clone, though this may also be associated with the development of graft versus host disease.

Treatment duration and treatment-free remission

Until recently, patients responding well to TKIs were told that therapy was lifelong but that those achieving stable major molecular responses were likely to be 'functionally cured' and expect to live a normal life span. However, data from the French 'Stop Imatinib' studyshow that approximately 40% of patient who had achieved complete molecular responses remained molecularly negative by Q-PCR after discontinuing imatinib for a median of 50 months. Further studies have confirmed these findings and suggest that a number of patients with particularly low levels of *BCR–ABL* transcripts may be able to discontinue treatment and remain in what is termed a 'treatment-free remission', although this continues to be evaluated as part of ongoing clinical trials.

Advanced-phase disease

A small number of patients may present with advanced-phase disease, though the majority of advanced-disease patients have progressed from CP due to an inadequate response to treatment. It is characterised by an increasing percentage of primitive blast cells in the marrow and the development of cytopenias and other symptoms. In 80% of patients, immunophenotyping of the blast cells confirms that they have arisen from the myeloid lineage (similar to acute myeloid leukaemia), whilst 20% of cases are lymphoblastic (Figure 5.8).

Despite the advances in treatment for CML, the prognosis from advanced-phase CML remains poor. Treatment with high-dose

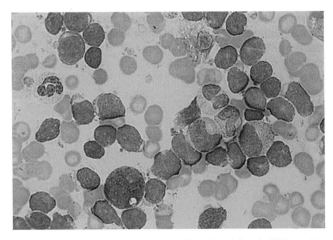

Figure 5.8 Peripheral blood appearance of a patient in lymphoid blast crisis. Source: *Post-Graduate Haematology* 5th edition, Fig 37.6.

TKIs alone may induce haematological and even cytogenetic responses in both myeloid and lymphoid blast crisis, but these responses are usually transient. The combination of TKIs and intensive chemotherapy further improves the response rate, and most patients who have achieved a response should be considered for an early allogeneic transplant, since this is the only known curative treatment. However, the overall survival following allogeneic transplantation for advanced-phase disease is <40% in most studies, due to the increased relapse rate.

Further reading

Baccarani M, Deininger MW, Rosti G *et al.* (2013) European LeukemiaNet recommendations for the management of chronic myeloid leukemia: 2013. *Blood*, **122**, 872–884.

Deininger M, Goldman JM and Melo JM (2000) The molecular biology of chronic myeloid leukemia. *Blood*, **96**, 3343–3356.

Deininger M, O'Brien SG, Guilhot F *et al.* (2009) International Randomized Study of Interferon vs. STI571 (IRIS) 8-year follow up: sustained survival and low risk for progression of events in patients with newly diagnosed chronic myeloid leukemia in chronic phase (CML-CP) treated with imatinib. *Blood*, **114**, 1126.

Jabbour E and Kantarjian H (2014) Chronic myeloid leukemia: 2014 update on diagnosis, monitoring, and management. *American Journal of Hematology*, **89**(5), 547–556.

Jabbour E, Branford S, Saglio G and Jones D (2011) Practical advice for determining the role of *BCR–ABL* mutations in guiding tyrosine kinase inhibitor therapy in patients with chronic myeloid leukemia. *Cancer*, **117**, 1800–1811.

Mahon FX, Réa D, Guilhot J *et al.* (2010) Discontinuation of imatinib in patients with chronic myeloid leukaemia who have maintained complete molecular remission for at least 2 years: the prospective, multicenter Stop Imatinib (STIM) trial. *Lancet Oncology*, **11**, 1029–1035.

CHAPTER 6

The Acute Leukaemias

John de Vos[1], Sandra Hassan[2] and Julia Sikorska[1]

[1] Royal Surrey County Hospital NHS Foundation Trust, Guildford, UK
[2] Queen's Hospital, BHR NHS Trust, Romford, UK

OVERVIEW

- Acute leukaemias develop as a consequence of acquired genetic abnormalities in haemopoietic stem cells.

- Acute leukaemias can be subdivided into acute myeloid leukaemia (AML) and acute lymphoblastic leukaemia (ALL).

- AML and ALL both present with symptoms of bone marrow failure caused by anaemia, neutropenia or thrombocytopenia.

- Chromosomal (cytogenetic) abnormalities define different biological subgroups of AML and ALL.

- Patient age, cytogenetic classification and response to initial chemotherapy are important factors allowing risk stratification.

- Treatment of both ALL and AML is initially with myelosuppressive chemotherapy.

- Allogeneic stem cell transplantation is reserved for patients predicted to have a poor outcome with chemotherapy alone.

Introduction

The acute leukaemias are malignant disorders of the bone marrow (haematopoietic system), with the white cell precursors as the cell of origin. The acquisition of distinct underlying genetic abnormalities in these haematopoietic stem cells or committed precursor cells leads to a proliferation of malignant cells, the leukaemic cells or 'blasts', causing normal haematopoiesis to be impaired. This leads to bone marrow failure. Clinically, patients therefore invariably present with symptoms of anaemia, thrombocytopenia or infections due to neutropenia (Table 6.1).

If this malignant transformation and subsequent proliferation occurs in precursors of lymphoid lineage this results in acute lymphoblastic leukaemia (ALL). If this transformation and proliferation occurs in myeloid precursors, then this results in acute myeloid leukaemia (AML).

The genetic abnormalities at the basis of the acute leukaemias frequently occur as the result of chromosomal translocations or the loss of chromosomal material. In addition, activating mutations in genes regulating cellular proliferation, such as tyrosine kinase genes, are commonly identified.

Table 6.1 Risk factors for the development of acute leukaemia.

The majority of cases of leukaemia have no apparent risk factors
Hereditary
Down's syndrome
Fanconi's anaemia
Bloom's syndrome
Klinefelter's syndrome
Wiskott–Aldrich syndrome
Ataxia telangiectasia
Osteogenesis imperfecta
Severe combined immunodeficiency
Neurofibromatosis type 1
Increased risk in siblings of affected child
Acquired
Carcinogen exposure
Previous chemotherapy treatment (DNA damaging)
Benzene
Radiation
Prior haematological disorder
Chronic myeloid leukaemia
Other myeloproliferative neoplasm (essential thrombocythaemia, polycythemia vera, myelofibrosis)
Myelodysplastic syndrome
Aplastic anaemia
Paroxysmal nocturnal haemoglobinuria

These abnormalities have become better understood during the last decade and are now incorporated in risk stratification of both ALL and AML. The identification of recognised abnormalities should now be standard practice and carries significant prognostic value. Identification is essential for accurate classification of the acute leukaemias (see later) and risk-adapted treatment.

In the past decades there has been a marked improvement in overall survival rates in patients presenting with acute leukaemia, most dramatically in childhood ALL. This progress has occurred as a result of both rigorous evaluation of chemotherapeutic drugs and supportive care in the setting of large-scale randomised studies, as well as incorporation of genetic abnormalities in risk stratification, risk-adapted treatment and remission monitoring. Identification of more and more molecular abnormalities holds the promise of possible future targets for new therapies.

ABC of Clinical Haematology, Fourth Edition. Edited by Drew Provan.
© 2018 John Wiley & Sons Ltd. Published 2018 by John Wiley & Sons Ltd.

Classification

The acute leukaemias are subdivided into AML and ALL. AML is a disease of myeloid progenitors (cells from which neutrophils, eosinophils, monocytes, basophils, megakaryocytes and erythrocytes are derived) and is characterised by the proliferation of myeloid blasts within the bone marrow and subsequently within the peripheral blood (Figure 6.1). ALL, by contrast, is a disease of lymphoid progenitors (immature lymphocytes), resulting in infiltration and proliferation of the bone marrow by lymphoid blasts (Figure 6.2).

Historically, the French–American–British classification was used to subdivide AML and ALL on the basis of morphological criteria. This was superseded by the World Health Organization classification, which incorporated morphological findings, as well as immunophenotypic and genetic/molecular abnormalities. The *WHO Classification of Tumours of Haematopoietic and Lymphoid Tissues* was updated in 2008 to include established subtypes of AML and ALL with recurrent genetic abnormalities.

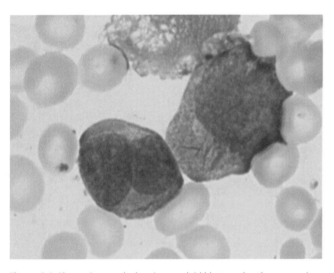

Figure 6.1 Photomicrograph showing myeloid blasts and pathognomonic Auer rod in patient with AML.

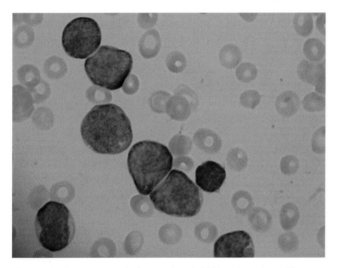

Figure 6.2 Photomicrograph showing lymphoid blasts in patient with ALL.

Epidemiology

ALL is the most common cancer of childhood. The highest incidence is seen in children 0–4 years of age (5.2 cases per 100 000 per year), falling to 1.9 cases per 100 000 per year in children 10–14 years of age. It is a much rarer leukaemia in adults, though there is a secondary rise in incidence in patients over the age of 40, but not to the levels seen in childhood. Generally, prognosis in childhood is much more favourable compared with ALL in adults.

AML is much rarer in childhood and much more common in adults, with an overall incidence of 3.4 per 100 000 per year, and nearly two-thirds of cases occurring in patients over the age of 60 years. Generally, prognosis in younger patients (<55 years) is much more favourable compared with AML in older patients.

The majority of cases of acute leukaemia are sporadic, although a number of factors associated with an increased risk of developing leukaemia have been identified (Table 6.1). Very rare familial cases have been described.

Clinical features of acute (myeloid and lymphoblastic) leukaemia

Acute leukaemias can present with a wide range of symptoms and signs, reflecting either as the direct result of bone marrow failure or infiltration of other organs with leukaemic blasts or the systemic consequences of advanced malignancy. Patients can simply present on the basis of a blood test or be very unwell. Acute leukaemia should be considered in the differential diagnosis of a number of common clinical presentations (Table 6.2). The features discussed in the following are seen in both AML and ALL with some differences highlighted.

Anaemia-related symptoms

Tiredness/fatigue, shortness of breath and pallor are common symptoms of anaemia commonly present at presentation.

Table 6.2 Differential diagnosis of acute leukaemia.

High white count/blasts on peripheral blood film due to other process
    'Leukaemoid reaction' (e.g. as seen in severe infection)
    Marrow infiltration by non-haematological cancers
    Chronic leukaemias
    Myeloproliferative neoplasms

Lymphadenopathy
    Lymphoma
    Non-haemopoietic malignancy
    Viral infection (e.g. infectious mononucleosis, HIV)
    Other infections (e.g. TB)
    Autoimmune disease

Hepatosplenomegaly
    Lymphoproliferative disease
    Myeloproliferative disease
    Storage disease
    Autoimmune disease
    Tropical disease

Myelodysplasia

Lymphoblastic lymphoma

Chronic leukaemias

Infection

Neutropenia (reduced neutrophil count) is very common at diagnosis, and results in an increased risk of both bacterial and fungal infections. Bacterial infection of the chest, throat, skin or perianal region is commonly seen and may be missed unless the relevant areas are carefully examined. Fungal infections most commonly present either as oral candidiasis or invasive intrapulmonary aspergillosis. Even if the neutrophil count appears normal, neutrophil function can often be poor, particularly in patients with a prior history of myelodysplastic syndrome in which neutrophils are usually dysfunctional ('functional neutropenia'). Patients presenting with acute leukaemia should therefore be considered neutropenic irrespective of their white cell count. Septicaemia is a common presentation of patients with acute leukaemia.

Bleeding

Bleeding can occur as a consequence of thrombocytopenia or abnormal coagulation. Spontaneous bruising, gingival bleeding, palatal and retinal haemorrhages, epistaxis, menorrhagia and prolonged bleeding after venepuncture are all relatively common. Acute promyelocytic leukaemia (APML, or 'AML M3'), a specific subtype of AML, typically presents with disseminated intravascular coagulation (DIC) with an associated marked thrombocytopenia. Serious bleeding in patients with APML at presentation is very common.

Infiltration

Leukaemic blast cells can infiltrate any organ. Infiltration of the meninges, resulting in headaches or cranial nerve palsies, is particularly common in ALL. Consequently, lumbar puncture is mandatory in newly diagnosed patients with ALL for both diagnostic and treatment purposes. Hepatosplenomegaly is frequently present at diagnosis in ALL, and mediastinal enlargement is well documented in T-cell ALL. ALL can also involve the testes, presenting with a painful testicular mass. These features are much less common in patients with AML. Bone pain is a direct consequence of bone marrow expansion, and is seen in both AML and ALL. Skin and gum infiltration occur more commonly in patients with AML.

Leucostasis

In patients presenting with acute leukaemia with high peripheral blood white cell counts, leucostasis can occur. This is rare but potentially fatal if not recognised. Symptoms of hyperviscosity, namely shortness of breath, visual disturbances, headaches and other neurological symptoms should raise the suspicion.

Diagnosis of acute (myeloid and lymphoblastic) leukaemia

A clinical suspicion will lead to the diagnostic tests outlined in the following. The investigations described are for both AML and ALL. Not all investigations might be required for all patients, keeping in mind not all patients will be fit for intensive and potentially curative treatment.

Full blood count

The blood count is nearly always abnormal in patients with acute leukaemia, and it is often the investigation that leads to the suspicion of the diagnosis of acute leukaemia in the first place. Patients with acute leukaemia commonly present with circulating leukaemic blasts in the peripheral blood, which are identified on a blood film. Commonly, there is an associated thrombocytopenia, neutropenia and anaemia. Mistakenly, people think that patients always present with raised white cell counts; though this is indeed a common presentation, many patients present with reduced white cell counts. Sometimes, no circulating blasts are present, but the cytopenias themselves might raise the suspicion for acute leukaemia.

Coagulation

The coagulation profile can be abnormal in patients presenting with acute leukaemia. DIC is often present in newly diagnosed patients with acute leukaemia and may result in life-threatening bleeding complications. DIC is a common finding secondary to sepsis, in itself a common presenting symptom, as well as potentially being directly triggered by the underlying leukaemia (as seen in APML; see earlier). Consequently, measurement of the platelet count, prothrombin time, activated partial thromboplastin time and fibrinogen are essential in all newly diagnosed patients and if abnormal require prompt correction and treatment of the underlying cause.

Biochemistry

Secondary changes can be found. Abnormal renal function can be seen secondary to hyperuricaemia (particularly with high white blood cell counts) and sepsis. Infiltration of the liver can cause abnormal liver function tests. Auto-tumour lysis in patients with high white cell counts or tumour lysis when treatment starts can lead to marked electrolyte disturbances that will require very close management and monitoring.

Bone marrow aspirate and trephine biopsy

A diagnosis of leukaemia can often be made from the full blood count and immunophenotyping on peripheral blood (see the following subsection), but a bone marrow aspiration and trephine remain essential for confirmation of diagnosis as well as for obtaining the correct samples for cytogenetic analysis and molecular studies. A trephine might not always be necessary, but if an aspirate fails (a 'dry tap') a trephine is recommended. Bone marrow aspirate results are often available on the same day as the procedure; they are generally performed and interpreted by haematologists.

Immunophenotyping

Leukaemic blasts aberrantly express antigens on their cell surface which can be identified via immunophenotyping. Distinct patterns of antigen expression permit accurate discrimination between myeloblasts and lymphoblasts, allowing confident distinction between AML and ALL. Immunophenotyping can be done both on the peripheral blood and on the bone marrow aspirate. Guidelines now recommend immunophenotyping results being available before commencing treatment, bar in life-threatening circumstances where emergency treatment can be commenced on the basis of the full blood count, blood film and/or bone marrow aspirate.

Cytogenetics and molecular studies

As mentioned earlier, distinct genetic and molecular abnormalities are present in many newly diagnosed patients with acute leukaemia. These abnormalities provide critically important risk stratification and prognostic information. They can often determine the course of treatment for a patient.

The identification of these abnormalities also provide markers for assessing response to treatment, and in many cases the persisting presence of genetic/molecular abnormalities after induction treatment will lead to a change in strategy and treatment.

- Three prognostic risk groups exist in AML patients based on cytogenetic examination at diagnosis. Karyotypic analysis is recommended in all patients undergoing intensive chemotherapy treatment.
  - Good risk group: patients with the chromosomal abnormalities t(8;21) (Figure 6.3), inv(16) or t(15;17) (Figure 6.4) have a good prognosis when treated with intensive chemotherapy alone.
  - Poor risk: generally patients with abnormalities of chromosomes 3, 5 or 7, or complex (four or more unrelated cytogenetic abnormalities) karyotypic abnormalities respond poorly to chemotherapy alone.
  - Standard risk: entities not classified as good or poor risk. These carry an intermediate prognosis.
- In AML, two molecular abnormalities have more recently modified risk stratification further in AML management. The FLT3 mutation is associated with a poor risk prognosis (irrespective of other cytogenetic abnormalities) and carries a high relapse risk. The NPM mutation carries a relatively favourable risk but can be negated by associated abnormalities.

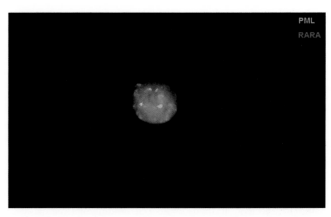

Figure 6.4 Fluorescence in-situ hybridisation examination in patient with APML demonstrating t(15;17).

Molecular analysis is now standard practice and should be recommended in all patients undergoing intensive chemotherapy treatment.

- In ALL, cytogenetics provide important prognostic information with the presence of the Philadelphia chromosome (t(9;22)) predicting poor long-term disease-free survival, whilst hyperdiploid karyotypes are associated with an improved outcome. In ALL, monitoring of cytogenetic abnormalities via minimal residual disease monitoring has been incorporated into treatment algorithms. If changes persist, treatment is escalated accordingly.

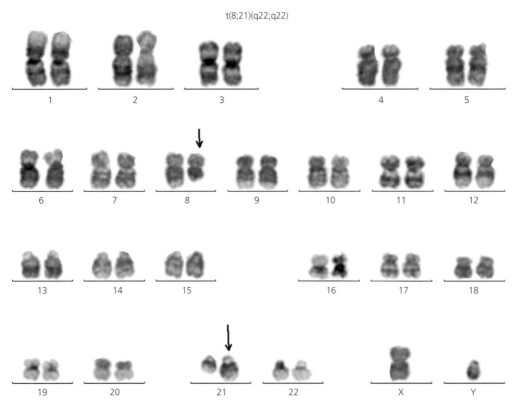

Figure 6.3 Karyotypic analysis in patient with AML associated with t(8;21).

Lumbar puncture

The presence of leukaemia in the central nervous system (CNS) should be suspected on the basis of clinical symptoms (headaches, visual disturbance, CNS symptoms). It is common at diagnosis and relapse in ALL but only rarely occurs in AML. Diagnosis is made on cerebrospinal fluid cytology. ALL treatment regimens routinely include administration of intrathecal chemotherapy (chemotherapy administered directly into the cerebrospinal fluid).

Principles of treatment

If untreated, acute leukaemia is invariably fatal. However, with intensive chemotherapy treatment it is a potentially curable disease. Both AML and ALL should be treated in specialised centres by a specialist multidisciplinary team. Table 6.3 lists the early principles of management.

At presentation the most important decision is whether or not a patient will be fit to undergo intensive chemotherapy treatment. The chemotherapy regimens for AML and ALL are intense and require prolonged hospital admissions. The patient's age, performance status, comorbidities and wishes need to be taken into account. Generally, an age cut-off of 60–70 years is used (slightly arbitrarily) above which intensive chemotherapy treatment might not be appropriate. Although not usually available immediately at diagnosis, cytogenetic studies can aid in this decision, and if possible it might be appropriate to withhold treatment until results are back in this group of patients. These decisions will need to be made by an experienced clinician who is used to looking after chemotherapy patients.

In elderly patients and patients not deemed fit for intensive chemotherapy, supportive management with blood product support or palliative chemotherapy regimens can be appropriate. The decision to treat or not to treat is complex and must be taken in careful consultation with the patient and their family, and in the context of the multidisciplinary team. In light of the toxicity of induction chemotherapy it is important to define patients in whom there is no realistic prospect of benefit from those patients who may expect a durable benefit.

Supportive care

Infection/septicaemia is the biggest risk in acute leukaemia patients undergoing treatment, and the threshold to start broad-spectrum antibiotics should be very low. An added risk is that patients will

Table 6.3 Principles of management of acute leukaemia.

- Management by specialist team
- Prompt clinical assessment and, where appropriate, institution of supportive care
- Exclusion of significant coagulopathy
- Rehydration and commencement of allopurinol (or rasburicase in patients to be at high risk of tumour lysis syndrome) in anticipation of treatment with chemotherapy
- Rapid diagnosis
- Discussion of diagnosis and treatment options with experienced clinician and clinical nurse specialist
- Review of diagnosis and treatment plan at multidisciplinary team meeting (may be *post hoc*)
- Swift institution of intensive chemotherapy
- Institution of CNS-directed chemotherapy where appropriate

Table 6.4 Supportive care.

- In-patient care in a specialist unit
- If patients are hypotensive, aggressive treatment of possible septic shock, including broad-spectrum antibiotics, aggressive fluid resuscitation and if necessary transfer to the intensive care unit are critical
- Placement of long-term central venous catheter
- Red cell transfusion to maintain haemoglobin >80 g/L
- Platelet transfusion to maintain platelet count $>10 \times 10^9$/L in patients unless patients are:
  - ○ febrile
  - ○ actively bleeding
  in which case maintain platelet count $>20 \times 10^9$/L
- Institution of broad-spectrum antibiotics in neutropenic patients with temperature >38.0 °C as per local guidelines

Table 6.5 Side-effects of chemotherapy.

Immediate
- Alopecia
- Nausea and vomiting
- Mucositis
- Hepatic dysfunction
- Haematological toxicity, including neutropenia and thrombocytopenia
- Peripheral neuropathy (e.g. vincristine)
- CNS toxicity (e.g. high-dose cytarabine)

Late
- Infertility
- Cardiomyopathy (anthracyclines)
- Pulmonary fibrosis
- Secondary malignancies, including myelodysplasia and leukaemia
- Growth failure
- Cognitive dysfunction
- Pulmonary fibrosis

invariably have indwelling central lines. Patients should receive antifungal and antiviral prophylaxis, and in some cases antibiotic prophylaxis, throughout. From presentation and during treatment, supportive care is essential in managing anaemia and thrombocytopenia. Transfusion support is vital throughout treatment. See also Table 6.4.

General principles of management

The initial aim of treatment is to achieve a complete remission, which is defined by the reduction of leukaemic blasts in the bone marrow to <5%. The initial cycle or block of treatment is therefore 'induction treatment'. If remission is achieved, further cycles or blocks of treatment ('consolidation') are given with the aim to maintain remission and reduce the relapse risk. Based on risk stratification, *some* patients will be recommended to have stem cell transplantation. Side effects of chemotherapy are listed in Table 6.5.

Specific management of acute myeloid leukaemia

Chemotherapy

Intensive chemotherapy with curative intent is given as an in-patient and is given in cycles. Each cycle (administration and recovery) will last 3–4 weeks. The first two cycles of chemotherapy are called induction treatment and routinely contain daunorubicin (anthracycline) and cytarabine. Complete remissions can be achieved in 70–80% of newly diagnosed adults using one or two cycles of induction chemotherapy. Risk stratification on the basis of age, white cell count at diagnosis and cytogenetics will lead to a risk-adapted approach to treatment. Low and standard-risk patients would continue with chemotherapy and would standardly have two more cycles of (consolidation) chemotherapy. There is a trend towards giving a total of three cycles of treatment in total, though data from large randomised controlled trials is eagerly awaited. In high-risk patients, consideration to stem cell transplantation should be given (see the following subsection).

APML, a specific subtype of leukaemia, is treated differently with a combination of an anthracycline and *all-trans*-retinoic acid, which is uniquely effective in this disease and has cure rates of around 90% of patients.

Role of stem cell transplantation

Allogeneic stem cell transplantation using a human leucocyte antigen (HLA) identical sibling or volunteer matched unrelated donor has the capacity to reduce the relapse rate and improve disease-free survival. Stem cell transplantation is reserved for patients with high-risk leukaemia based on age, presenting white cell count and cytogenetic studies. Some patients with standard-risk cytogenetics are recommended to have stem cell transplantation, but this should be decided within the context of a multidisciplinary team and the final decision made by an experienced clinician in conjunction with the patient. Stem cell transplantation is not indicated in patients with good-risk cytogenetics, as outcome with chemotherapy alone is favourable. Stem cell transplantation should occur once the patient is in remission and should follow on from their induction chemotherapy or from their consolidation chemotherapy.

The main problem of stem cell transplantation has always been the associated toxicity, morbidity and mortality. This has markedly reduced over the last decade with much improved supportive care and the introduction of reduced-intensity allogeneic stem cell transplantation (or 'mini'-transplants). The full myelo-ablative transplant regimens only continue to be used in paediatric patients and young adults. Reduced-intensity transplantation has led to the upper age limit for patients being increased to 65–70 years, a remarkable breakthrough that has markedly improved outcomes for older patients undergoing intensive treatment for AML.

Management of relapse

Despite intensive treatment and stem cell transplantation, relapsed AML occurs in a significant proportion of AML patients. Adverse prognostic features at diagnosis (high white cell count, older age, poor risk cytogenetics) significantly increase this risk. If patients are fit enough re-induction treatment ('salvage' treatment) and subsequent stem cell transplantation represents the only curative treatment option for these patients. In patients whose duration of first remission is less than one year, long term survival rates even with intensive treatment and stem cell transplantation are less than 10% and this information is clearly important when coming to a decision with the patient whether to proceed with treatment or opt for supportive/palliative measures.

Specific management of acute lymphoblastic leukaemia

Chemotherapy

Intensive chemotherapy with a curative intent is the mainstay of treatment. The first block of treatment is given with the aim to induce a complete remission ('induction'), and further treatment blocks are given as consolidation. Cure rates are high in children, but very poor in adults. This is directly related to the cytogenetics changes seen in the different age groups. The treatment principles in ALL are the same as in patients receiving treatment for AML, though there are significant differences:

1 Apart from chemotherapy agents such as anthracyclines and cytarabine, different drugs include vincristine and L-asparaginase, two drugs highly active in ALL treatment.
2 Patients with ALL receive treatment directed at treating and/or preventing CNS infiltration by leukaemia. ALL patient receive regular intrathecal administration of chemotherapy agents, as well as administration of high-dose methotrexate (with the capability of crossing the blood–brain barrier if given in high enough doses), and in some cases cranio-spinal radiotherapy.
3 In addition to the aforementioned drugs, imatinib (Glivec®) is highly active in patients with Philadelphia-positive (Ph+) ALL and is an important addition to conventional chemotherapy in this subgroup of patients. Ph + ALL is more common in adults and generally carries a poor prognosis.
4 Patients with ALL receive maintenance treatment (2 years for women/girls, 3 years for men/boys) with oral drugs including 6-mercaptopurine and methotrexate. Maintenance treatment has been shown to improve overall survival in adults and children with ALL.

Role of stem cell transplantation

As in AML, allogeneic stem cell transplantation using an HLA identical sibling or a volunteer matched unrelated donor has the capacity to reduce the relapse rate and improve disease-free survival.

In children, ALL generally carries a favourable prognosis, relating to the favourable cytogenetic abnormalities seen in this group. Stem cell transplantation is therefore generally only reserved for patients at relapse and not used in frontline management, though exceptions (as always in medicine) exist.

In adults, ALL carries a poor prognosis, relating to the poor-risk cytogenetics seen in this group of patients (including Ph + ALL), and stem cell transplantation is generally considered in these patients once remission after first-line treatment is achieved. Exceptions again exist.

Novel therapies

Despite great advances in the understanding of the pathogenesis and pathophysiology of AML and ALL, as well as the hope that discovered genetic abnormalities might be targets for specific treatment, not many new drugs have made it through the trial stages. The success of imatinib (Glivec®) in patients with chronic myeloid leukaemia has led to the hope that it may be possible in the future to identify similar targets in AML and ALL. However, though some drugs are in use they have not as yet fulfilled their promise.

Azacitidine, a cytosine nucleoside analogue and DNA hypomethylating agent, has been successfully used in patients with myelodysplastic syndrome, and a use in non-proliferating AML unfit for intensive treatment is currently in clinical trials.

There clearly remains a need for the development of new treatments in AML and ALL.

Further reading

Curran E and Stock W. (2015) How I treat acute lymphoblastic leukaemia in older adolescents and young adults. *Blood*, **125**, 3702–3710.

Fielding A (2010) How I treat Philadelphia chromosome-positive acute lymphoblastic leukaemia. *Blood*, **116**, 3409–3417.

Grimwade D, Walker H, Oliver F *et al.* (1998) The importance of diagnostic cytogenetics on outcome in AML: analysis of 1,612 patients entered into the MRC AML 10 trial. *Blood*, **92**(7), 2322–2333.

Grimwade D, Hills RK, Moorman AV *et al.* (2010) Refinement of cytogenetic classification in acute myeloid leukaemia: determination of prognostic significance of rare recurring chromosomal abnormalities in 5876 younger adult patients treated in the United Kingdom Medical Research Council Trials. *Blood*, **116**(3), 354–365.

Pui CH and Evans WE (2006) Treatment of acute lymphoblastic leukemia. *New England Journal of Medicine*, **354**(2), 166–178.

Rowe JM and Tallman MS (2010) How I treat acute myeloid leukaemia. *Blood*, **116**, 3147–3156.

Swerdlow SH, Campo E, Harris NL *et al.* (eds) (in press) *WHO Classification of Tumours of Haematopoietic and Lymphoid Tissues*, WHO Classification of Tumours, revised 4th edition, Vol. 2, IARC Press, Lyon.

Tallman MS and Altman JK (2009) How I treat acute promyelocytic leukaemia. *Blood*, **114**, 5126–5135.

Tauro S, Craddock C, Peggs, K *et al.* (2005) Allogeneic stem cell transplantation using a reduced intensity conditioning (RIC) regimen has the capacity to produce durable remissions and long term disease free survival in patients with high risk acute myeloid leukemia (AML) and myelodysplasia (MDS). *Journal of Clinical Oncology*, **23**, 9387–9393.

CHAPTER 7

Platelet Disorders

Marie A. Scully[1] and R. J. Liesner[2]

[1] Department of Haematology, University College London Hospitals NHS Trust, Cardiometabolic Programme-NIHR UCLH/ UCL BRC, London, UK
[2] Great Ormond Street Hospital, London, UK

OVERVIEW

- Platelets are produced from bone marrow megakaryocytes.

- They are important in the formation of platelet plugs during normal haemostasis.

- Surface glycoprotein receptors on platelets are important in platelet–platelet and platelet–endothelial cell adhesion.

- Release of platelet contents from storage organelles within platelets is important in platelet aggregation.

- Surface phospholipid of platelets is important in interaction and activation of clotting factors in the coagulation pathway.

- Congenital platelet disorders are divided into:
  - platelet production (e.g. thrombocytopenia with absent radii syndrome, Wiskott–Aldrich syndrome);
  - functional platelet abnormalities (e.g. Bernard–Soulier syndrome, Glanzmann thrombasthenia).

- Acquired platelet abnormalities can be divided into:
  - bone marrow failure (e.g. aplastic anaemia, leukaemic bone marrow infiltration);
  - peripheral consumption (e.g. immune thrombocytopenia, post-transfusion purpura, neonatal alloimmune thrombocytopenia, thrombotic thrombocytopenic purpura);
  - a full bleeding history, drug history and review of the peripheral blood film are of primary importance in the differential diagnosis;
  - increasingly, molecular diagnosis is useful in congenital abnormalities.

- Available treatments depend on the diagnosis:
  - platelet concentrates (contraindicated in thrombotic thrombocytopenic purpura);
  - intravenous immunoglobulin;
  - tranexamic acid;
  - desmopressin;
  - recombinant factor VIIa;
  - bone marrow transplantation.

Platelets are small anucleate cells produced predominantly by the bone marrow megakaryocytes as a result of budding of the cytoplasmic membrane. Megakaryocytes are derived from the haemopoietic stem cell, which is stimulated to differentiate to mature megakaryocytes under the influence of various cytokines, including thrombopoietin. Platelets play a key role in securing primary haemostasis.

Once released from the bone marrow, young platelets are trapped in the spleen for up to 36 h before entering the circulation, where they have a primary haemostatic role. Their normal lifespan is 7–10 days, and the normal platelet count for all age groups is $(150–450) \times 10^9$/L. The mean platelet diameter is 1–2 μm, and the normal range for cell volume (mean platelet volume) is 8–11 fL. Although platelets are non-nucleated cells, those that have recently been released from the bone marrow contain RNA and are known as reticulated platelets. They normally represent 8–16% of the total count, and they indirectly indicate the state of marrow production.

Normal haemostasis

The platelet membrane contains integral glycoproteins essential in the initial events of adhesion and aggregation, leading to the formation of the platelet plug during haemostasis (Figure 7.1).

Glycoprotein receptors react with aggregating agents, such as collagen on the damaged vascular endothelial surface and fibrinogen and von Willebrand factor (VWF), to facilitate platelet–platelet and platelet–endothelial cell adhesion. The major glycoproteins are the Ib/IX complex, the main binding protein of which is VWF, and IIb/IIIa, which specifically binds fibrinogen. Storage organelles within the platelet include the 'dense' granules, which contain nucleotides, calcium and serotonin, and α granules containing fibrinogen, VWF, platelet-derived growth factor and many other clotting factors. Following adhesion, the platelets are stimulated to release the contents of their granules, essential for platelet

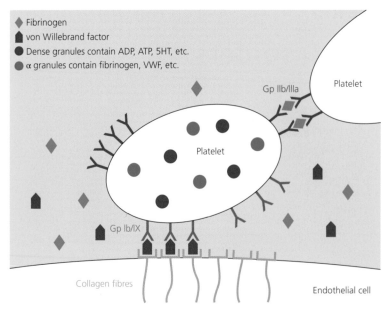

Figure 7.1 Normal platelet function.

aggregation. The platelets also provide an extensive phospholipid surface for the interaction and activation of clotting factors in the coagulation pathway.

Congenital abnormalities

Congenital abnormalities of platelets can be divided into disorders of platelet production and those of platelet function. All are very rare. In general, they cause moderate to severe bleeding problems. Increasingly, the molecular basis for these disorders has been characterised and therefore can usually be used as a diagnostic tool, and may facilitate antenatal diagnosis.

Fanconi anaemia

Fanconi anaemia is an autosomal recessive preleukaemic condition, which often presents as thrombocytopenia with skeletal or genitourinary abnormalities. The cardinal laboratory feature is abnormal chromosomal fragility. The majority of cases are caused by abnormalities in one of three genes, *FANCA*, *FANCC* and *FANCG*, resulting in inefficient repair of damaged DNA. The condition can be cured with bone marrow transplantation.

Thrombocytopenia with absent radii

Thrombocytopenia with absent radii syndrome presents with the pathognomonic sign of bilateral absent radii (Figure 7.2) and with severe ($<10 \times 10^9$/L) neonatal thrombocytopenia, although this often starts to improve after the first year of life. Mutations are in *RBM8A* (chromosome 1q21). This should be distinguished from amegakaryocytic thrombocytopenia, another leukaemia predisposition syndrome, in which severe neonatal thrombocytopenia is present with orthopaedic or neurological abnormalities in 10–30% of children. The underlying genetic abnormality, located to the *c-MPL* gene on chromosome 1, affects the thrombopoietin receptor.

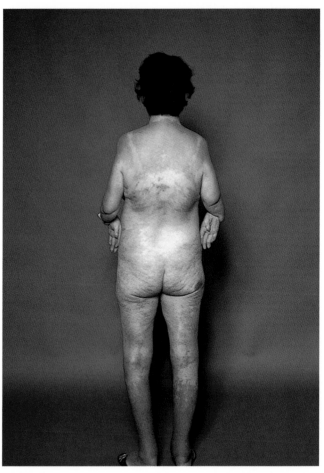

Figure 7.2 Amegakaryocytic thrombocytopenia with absent radii syndrome.

Wiskott–Aldrich syndrome

This is an X-linked disorder with a triad of thrombocytopenia, eczema and T-cell immunodeficiency. The platelet count is usually

$(20–100) \times 10^9$/L, and the platelets are small and functionally abnormal. The diagnosis can be confirmed by analysis of the *WAS* gene (Xp11). Like Fanconi anaemia, this condition can only be cured with bone marrow transplantation.

MYH9-related thrombocytopenias

MYH9-related thrombocytopenias, including the May–Hegglin anomaly, are autosomal dominant conditions associated with macro-thrombocytopenia (Figure 7.3). The genetic abnormality is in the *MYH9* gene, located on chromosome 22. Variants of Alport syndrome are also characterised by giant platelets, associated with progressive hereditary nephritis and deafness.

Disorders of the surface membrane

Disorders of the surface membrane are characterised by absence or abnormalities of platelet membrane glycoproteins, resulting in defective platelet adhesion and/or aggregation. These include

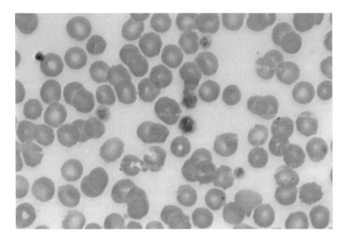

Figure 7.3 Giant granular platelets in peripheral blood film as seen in Bernard–Soulier syndrome or May–Hegglin anomaly.

Bernard–Soulier syndrome, an autosomal recessive condition, with macrothrombocytopenia and a lack of VWF-dependent platelet agglutination caused by mutations within the genes that encode for the glycoprotein (Gp)Ib/IX/V complex (Figure 7.4). Glanzmann thrombasthenia is associated with abnormalities of the GpIIb/IIIa receptor complex which results in a functional deficiency but with a normal platelet count. In platelet-type von Willebrand disease, spontaneous binding of plasma VWF to enlarged platelets results from mutations of GpIbα (Figure 7.4).

Platelet storage pool diseases

Deficiencies in either the α or dense granules cause poor secondary platelet aggregation. Absence of α granules in grey platelet syndrome, an autosomal dominant inherited condition, results in large, pale platelets on blood films. It results from mutations in *NBEAL2* gene on chromosome 3.

Other conditions

There are also a variety of further specific surface membrane defects and internal enzyme abnormalities, which, although difficult to define, can cause troublesome chronic bleeding problems.

Acquired abnormalities

Decreased production of platelets

Decreased platelet production caused by suppression or failure of the bone marrow is the commonest cause of thrombocytopenia. In aplastic anaemia, leukaemia and marrow infiltration, and after chemotherapy, thrombocytopenia is usually associated with a failure of red and white cell production, but may be an isolated finding secondary to drug toxicity (penicillamine, cotrimoxazole), alcohol or viral infection (human immunodeficiency virus, infectious mononucleosis). Viral infection is the most common cause of mild transient thrombocytopenia (Box 7.1).

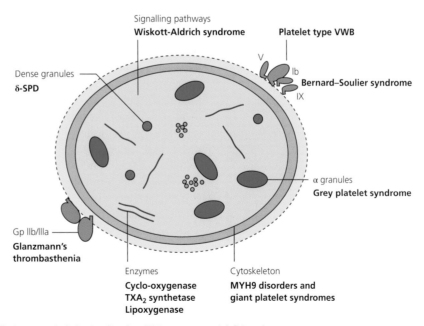

Figure 7.4 Site of abnormality in congenital platelet disorders (SPD: storage pool deficiency).

Box 7.1 **Acquired disorders of reduced platelet production due to bone marrow failure/replacement.**

- Drug induced
- Leukaemia
- Metastatic tumour
- Aplastic anaemia
- Myelodysplasia
- Cytotoxic drugs
- Radiotherapy
- Associated with infection
- Megaloblastic anaemia

Increased consumption of platelets

Increased platelet consumption may be due to immune or non-immune mechanisms.

Immune thrombocytopenia

Immune thrombocytopenia is a relatively common disorder and is the most frequent cause of an isolated thrombocytopenia without anaemia or neutropenia. In adults, it often presents insidiously, most frequently in women aged 15–50 years, and can be associated with other autoimmune diseases, in particular systemic lupus erythematosus or the primary antiphospholipid syndrome. In children, the onset is more acute and often follows a viral infection. The autoantibody produced is usually immunoglobulin G, directed against antigens on the platelet membrane. Antibody-coated platelets are removed by the reticuloendothelial system, reducing the lifespan of the platelets to a few hours. The platelet count can vary from $<5 \times 10^9$/L to near normal. The severity of bleeding is less than that seen with comparable degrees of thrombocytopenia in bone marrow failure, owing to the predominance of young, larger and functionally superior platelets (Figures 7.5 and 7.6, Box 7.2).

Post-transfusion purpura

Post-transfusion purpura is a rare complication of blood transfusion. It presents with severe thrombocytopenia 7–10 days after the transfusion and usually occurs in multiparous women who are negative for the human platelet antigen (HPA)1a. Antibodies to

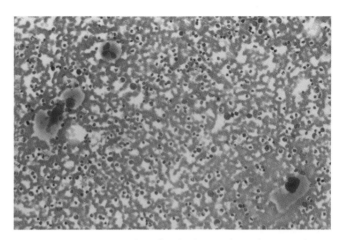

Figure 7.6 Bone marrow aspirate showing increased megakaryocytes in immune thrombocytopenia.

Box 7.2 **Disorders with increased consumption of platelets.**

- Disorders with immune mechanism
- Autoimmune: immune thrombocytopenia
- Alloimmune: post-transfusion purpura, neonatal alloimmune thrombocytopenia
- Infection associated: infectious mononucleosis, human immuno-deficiency virus, malaria
- Drug induced: heparin, penicillin, quinine, sulphonamides, rifampicin
- Thrombotic thrombocytopenic purpura/haemolytic uraemic syndrome
- Hypersplenism and splenomegaly
- Disseminated intravascular coagulation (DIC)
- Massive transfusion

HPA1a develop and, in some way, this alloantibody is responsible for the immune destruction of autologous (patient's own) platelets.

Neonatal alloimmune thrombocytopenia

Neonatal alloimmune thrombocytopenia is similar to haemolytic disease of the newborn except that the antigenic stimulus comes from platelet-specific antigens rather than red-cell antigens. In 80% of cases the antigen is HPA1a, and mothers who are negative for this antigen (about 5% of the population) or HPA5b form antibodies when sensitised by a fetus positive for the antigen. Fetal platelet destruction results from transplacental passage of these antibodies, and severe bleeding, including intracranial haemorrhage, can occur *in utero* or within the first few weeks of life. Firstborns are frequently affected, and successive pregnancies are equally or more affected.

Heparin-induced thrombocytopenia

Heparin-induced thrombocytopenia occurs during unfractionated heparin therapy in up to 5% of patients, but is less frequently associated with low molecular weight heparins. It may become manifest when arterial or venous thrombosis occurs during a fall in the platelet count and is thought to be due to the formation of antibodies to

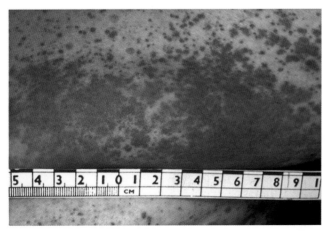

Figure 7.5 Spontaneous skin purpura in severe immune thrombocytopenia.

heparin that are bound to platelet factor 4, a platelet granule protein. The immune complexes activate platelets and endothelial cells, resulting in thrombocytopenia. Heparin-induced thrombocytopenia carries an appreciable morbidity and mortality, especially from resulting thrombosis, if the diagnosis is delayed.

Thrombotic thrombocytopenic purpura

The hallmarks of thrombotic thrombocytopenic purpura are thrombocytopenia and microangiopathic haemolytic anaemia with clinical symptoms affecting any organ, but primarily manifesting as neurological symptoms, resulting from microvascular thrombosis. The condition is associated with deficiency of ADAMTS 13, a metalloprotease enzyme responsible for cleaving the ultra-high molecular weight multimers of VWF. The condition is suspected clinically by thrombocytopenia, red cell fragmentation on the blood film and a reticulocytosis. The demonstration of an abnormal pattern of von Willebrand multimers makes the diagnosis highly likely, and the complete absence of the cleaving protease caused by an inhibitory antibody can be proven in some specialised laboratories (Figure 7.7).

Microangiopathic thrombocytopenia

Microangiopathic thrombocytopenia includes disorders such as preeclampsia or HELLP (*h*aemolysis, *e*levated *l*iver enzymes, *l*ow *p*latelets) syndrome in pregnancy, haemolytic uraemic syndrome, DIC and catastrophic antiphospholipid syndrome. The blood films may be similar in all these disorders, with thrombocytopenia, anaemia and fragmented red blood cells.

Disseminated intravascular coagulation

DIC usually occurs in critically ill patients as a result of catastrophic activation of the coagulation pathway, often due to sepsis. Widespread platelet consumption occurs, causing thrombocytopenia.

Massive blood transfusion

In patients with life-threatening bleeding, transfusion of 8–10 units of red blood cells without replacing clotting factors or platelets may result in prolonged clotting screen and thrombocytopenia.

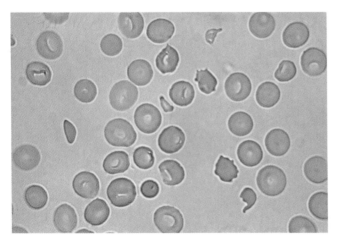

Figure 7.7 Red cell fragmentation in patient who presented with confusion and lethargy in whom thrombotic thrombocytopenic purpura was diagnosed. She responded well to large-volume plasma exchange for 1 week.

> Box 7.3 **Causes of acquired platelet dysfunction.**
>
> - Aspirin and non-steroidal anti-inflammatory agents
> - Penicillins and cephalosporins
> - Uraemia
> - Ethanol
> - Liver disease
> - Myeloproliferative disorders
> - Myeloma
> - Cardiopulmonary bypass
> - Fish oils

Massive splenomegaly

The spleen normally pools about a third of the platelet mass, but in massive splenomegaly this can increase up to 90%, resulting in apparent thrombocytopenia.

Drugs

Aspirin, non-steroidal anti-inflammatory agents and glycoprotein IIb/IIIa antagonists are the most common causes of acquired platelet dysfunction (Box 7.3). For this reason, aspirin and the IIb/IIIa antagonists are used therapeutically as antiplatelet agents. Aspirin acts by irreversibly inhibiting cyclo-oxygenase activity in the platelet, resulting in impairment of the granule release reaction and defective aggregation. The effects of a single dose of aspirin last for the lifetime of the platelet (7–10 days). Recently, clopidogrel, a thienopyridine derivative, has been introduced as an oral antiplatelet agent that inhibits adenosine diphosphate binding to the platelet membrane and is useful in patients who are intolerant or resistant to aspirin. It is becoming widely used as a prophylactic agent for myocardial ischaemia and related coronary syndromes.

Bleeding in uraemic patients

Bleeding most commonly results from defects in platelet adhesion or aggregation, although thrombocytopenia, severe anaemia with packed cell volume <20% or coagulation defects can also contribute.

Essential (primary) thrombocytosis and reactive (secondary) thrombocytosis

In these conditions, the platelet count is raised above the upper limit of normal. A wide range of disorders can cause a raised platelet count ($>800 \times 10^9$/L), but patients are normally asymptomatic, except in essential thrombocytosis, when excessive spontaneous bleeding may develop when the count exceeds 1000×10^9/L. Antiplatelet drugs can be useful to prevent thrombosis in high-risk patients; for example, postoperatively. Some myelodysplastic syndromes may be complicated by an acquired storage pool-type platelet disorder (Box 7.4).

History and examination of patients

Abnormal bleeding associated with thrombocytopenia or abnormal platelet function is characterised by spontaneous skin purpura and ecchymoses, mucous membrane bleeding and protracted bleeding after trauma. Prolonged nosebleeds can occur, particularly in children, and menorrhagia or post-partum haemorrhage is common in women. Rarely, subconjunctival, retinal, gastrointestinal,

Box 7.4 **Thrombocytosis.**

- Essential (primary) thrombocytosis
- Reactive (secondary) thrombocytosis
- Infection
- Malignant disease
- Acute and chronic inflammatory diseases
- Pregnancy
- Post-splenectomy
- Iron deficiency
- Haemorrhage

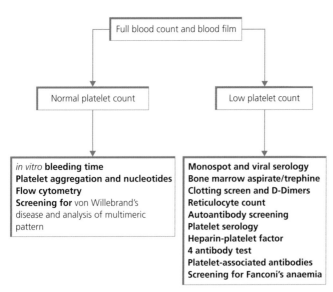

Figure 7.8 Investigation of suspected platelet disorder.

genitourinary and intracranial bleeds may occur. In thrombocytopenic patients, severe spontaneous bleeding is unusual with a platelet count $\geq 20 \times 10^9$/L, unless there is associated platelet dysfunction.

Investigations

The investigations in a suspected platelet disorder will depend on the presentation and history in each patient. If the bleeding is severe, the patient may need urgent hospital referral for prompt evaluation, diagnosis and treatment, which may entail blood product support. All patients should have a full blood count, coagulation and biochemical screen, and then further investigations depending on the results of these. A thorough review of the blood film can help in the diagnosis or exclusion of many disorders associated with thrombocytopenia (Figure 7.8).

Thrombocytopenia can be artefactual and due to platelet clumping or a blood clot in the sample, which should be excluded in all cases. The skin bleeding time, which is invasive, variable and not reliable in screening mild platelet disorders, has been replaced by devices that perform an *in vitro* bleeding time on small volumes of citrated blood and simulate platelet function in a high shear rate situation. The sensitivity of these devices for all platelet disorders is still under investigation.

Box 7.5 **Treatment of platelet disorders.**

Congenital disorders
- Platelet transfusions (leucodepleted, human leucocyte antigen compatible and irradiated)
- Desmopressin
- Tranexamic acid
- Recombinant factor VIIa
- Bone marrow transplantation

Acquired disorders

Bone marrow failure
- Platelet transfusions if platelet count $<10 \times 10^9$/L

Immune thrombocytopenia (adults)
- Prednisolone
- Intravenous immunoglobulin
- Anti-D immunoglobulin
- Rituximab
  - mycophenolate
  - thrombopoietin-receptor agonists
- Splenectomy

Post-transfusion purpura
- Intravenous immunoglobulin
- Plasma exchange
- Avoid platelet transfusions

Heparin-induced thrombocytopenia
- Anticoagulation but without heparin
- Avoid platelet transfusions

Thrombotic thrombocytopenic purpura
- Large-volume plasma exchange
- Aspirin when platelets $>50 \times 10^9$/L
- Avoid platelet transfusions

Disseminated intravascular coagulation
- Treat underlying cause
- Fresh frozen plasma
- Platelet transfusion
- Cryoprecipitate

Hypersplenism
- Splenectomy if severe

Platelet function disorders
- Platelet transfusion
- Desmopressin (occasionally of use, e.g. in uraemia)
- Tranexamic acid

Management

All serious bleeding due to a platelet disorder needs haematological assessment and treatment. Mild or trivial bleeding due to a transient postviral thrombocytopenia or aspirin ingestion needs no active treatment and can be managed on an outpatient basis (Box 7.5).

Congenital disorders

A neonate or small infant with bleeding must be referred for evaluation as the inherited bleeding disorders (e.g. haemophilia or von Willebrand disease) and platelet disorders can present at a very young age.

Severe bleeding episodes in all the congenital thrombocytopenias and platelet function disorders require filtered human leucocyte antigen-compatible platelet transfusions to secure haemostasis, although, in minor episodes in the milder dysfunctional syndromes, desmopressin (1-deamino-8-D-arginine vasopressin) given intravenously or intranasally with antifibrinolytics (tranexamic acid) may be sufficient. Recombinant factor VIIa (Novoseven®; Novartis) may be of use in the treatment or prevention of bleeding in a minority of rare bleeding disorders and is licensed for use in patients with Glanzmann thrombasthenia who have antibodies to the missing glycoprotein. This avoids exposure to blood products, but it is expensive and the response is variable. Bone marrow transplantation can potentially offer a cure in a number of these conditions.

Acquired disorders

In thrombocytopenia due to bone marrow failure or marrow infiltration (e.g. leukaemia or cancer), prophylactic platelet transfusions are given to keep the platelet count above $10 \times 10^9/L$, although the threshold is higher in infected or bleeding patients or to cover invasive procedures.

In childhood immune thrombocytopenia, spontaneous recovery is common, and treatment, such as corticosteroids or intravenous immunoglobulin, is given only if there are bleeding manifestations. In adults, the condition rarely remits without treatment and is more likely to become chronic. Initial treatment is either prednisolone 1 mg/kg daily (80% of cases remit), intravenous immunoglobulin (0.4 g/kg for 5 days or 1 g/kg for 2 days) or both. In refractory patients, splenectomy has a 60–70% chance of long-term cure, although the use of rituximab, an anti-CD20 monoclonal antibody, has proven equally effective without the need for surgical intervention. Other potential therapies include azathioprine, mycophenolate, high-dose dexamethasone and thrombopoietin-receptor agonists.

Patients in whom heparin-induced thrombocytopenia is suspected are often inpatients with ongoing thrombosis and may have complex medical problems. It is essential to stop heparin and treat thrombosis with other anticoagulants; further use of heparins should be avoided. Warfarin, synthetic heparinoids or direct oral anticoagulants can be used. Platelet transfusions are contraindicated in heparin-induced thrombocytopenia and in thrombotic thrombocytopenic purpura. If the latter is suspected clinically and on the basis of laboratory tests, large-volume plasma exchange should be started immediately and continued daily until substantial clinical improvement occurs and all the results of haematological tests have normalised. Aspirin can be started once the platelet count is $>50 \times 10^9/L$.

With DIC, it is essential to treat the underlying cause in addition to aggressive replacement of depleted clotting factors and platelets with blood products. In patients requiring massive blood transfusion, replacement with fresh frozen plasma (15 mL/kg) and a pool of platelets should be given with every 8–10 units of red cells received.

In pronounced bleeding or risk of bleeding due to the acquired disorders of platelet function, platelets usually have to be transfused to provide normally functioning platelets, although desmopressin and tranexamic acid can also be of value. Usually, treatment may only be necessary to cover surgical procedures or major haemorrhage.

Further reading

Hardisty RM (2000) Platelet functional disorders. In *Pediatric Hematology*, 2nd edn (eds J Lilleyman, I Hann and V Blanchette), Churchill Livingstone, London, chapter 24.

Nurden AT (2005) Qualitative disorders of platelets and megakaryocytes. *Journal of Thrombosis and Haemostasis*, **3**, 1773–1782.

Rendu F and Brohard-Bohn B (2001) The platelet release reaction: granules' constituents, secretion and functions. *Platelets*, **12**, 261–273.

Shapiro AP (2000) Platelet function disorders. *Haemophilia*, **6**, 120–127.

Siddiqui MAA and Scott LJ (2005) Recombinant factor VIIa (Eptacog alfa). A review of its use in congenital or acquired haemophilia and other congenital bleeding disorders. *Drugs*, **65**, 1161–1177.

Smith OP (2000) Inherited and congenital thrombocytopenia. In *Pediatric Hematology*, 2nd edn, (eds J Lilleyman, I Hann and V Blanchette), Churchill Livingstone, London, chapter 21.

CHAPTER 8

Myelodysplastic Syndromes

Ghulam J. Mufti and Robin Dowse

Haematological Medicine, King's College Hospital NHS Foundation Trust, Hambleden Wing, London, UK

OVERVIEW

- Myelodysplasia results in cytopenias, especially anaemia, with an increased risk of transformation to acute myeloid leukaemia.
- It is a disease particularly affecting the elderly.
- Prognosis is related to the cytogenetics of the malignant clone, the percentage of bone marrow blasts and the number of cytopenias.
- Treatment ranges from supportive care with blood products, immunotherapy and chemotherapy to allogeneic bone marrow transplantation, depending on the age and fitness of the patient, and the severity of the myelodysplasia.
- New promising agents include lenalidomide and azacitidine.

Introduction

Myelodysplastic syndromes (MDSs) are a heterogeneous group of acquired haemopoietic stem cell disorders characterised by

- ineffective haematopoiesis leading to cytopenias
- dysplasia in one or more myeloid cell lineages dependent on stage and disease subtype
- variable predilection for transformation to acute myeloid leukaemia (AML).

An MDS is predominantly a disease of the elderly, with an annual incidence of 4 per 100 000 population, rising to >30 per 100 000 in those over the age of 70 years.

Pathogenesis

Despite many advances, the exact pathogenesis of MDSs is not yet fully understood. In brief, the main insult is believed to be due to an acquired genetic or epigenetic abnormality of the bone marrow haemopoietic stem cells inducing genomic instability, and predisposition to further mutations. However, the initiating events remain uncertain. In cases with a therapy-related MDS (t-MDS) the disease follows ionising radiation, environmental toxins (such as pesticides and solvents) and chemotherapy (particularly after alkylating agents).

Genetic mutations

The acquisition of further mutations favours selection of a dysplastic clone due to a proliferative advantage, usually via upregulation of multiple pro-survival and cell cycle pathways. Additionally, acquisition of certain mutations may cause impaired differentiation (e.g. *RUNX1* mutations), altered ribosomal function (e.g. *RPS14* mutations in deletion 5q syndrome) or deregulated apoptosis (e.g. *cMyc* mutations). Mutations may also induce alterations in epigenetic regulation; for example, in histone modification, DNA methylation patterns and microRNA expression. Increasingly, analysis of the somatic mutations present in an MDS provides a useful adjunct to other investigations and predicts prognosis and response to treatment (Table 8.1).

Deregulation of immune processes

The higher incidence of autoimmune disease seen in those with an MDS suggests that immune deregulation plays an important role in disease pathogenesis. Moreover, the overlap between aplastic anaemia and hypoplastic MDS further supports this concept. T-cell-mediated inhibition of haematopoiesis either via upregulation of cytotoxic T cells or reduction of T-helper cells coupled with natural killer cell

Table 8.1 Examples of mutations seen in MDSs.

Category	Examples	Morphological/clinical effect
Epigenetic modification	EZH2	Poor prognosis
	ASXL1	Poor prognosis
	DNMT3A	Poor prognosis
	TET2	Increased response to hypomethylating agents
	IDH2	Poor prognosis
Spliceosome mutations	SRSF2	Poor prognosis
	SF3B1	Ring sideroblasts, good prognosis
	U2AF1	
Transcription factors	RUNX1	Poor prognosis
Oncogenes	NRAS	Increased marrow blast proportion
	TP53	Poor response to conventional chemotherapy

ABC of Clinical Haematology, Fourth Edition. Edited by Drew Provan.

dysfunction, and augmented pro-inflammatory cytokines such as tumour necrosis factor α or interferon γ all contribute to immune dysregulation.

Abnormal stem cell environment

Increasing evidence suggests that the bone marrow micro-environment contributes to maintenance of the abnormal stem cell clones and disease progression. For example, mesenchymal stem and progenitor cells can induce altered haematopoietic–stromal interactions as can abnormal macrophages, monocytes and myeloid-derived suppressor cells.

Spliceosome mutations

When mRNA is formed, non-coding regions (introns) are removed and the coding regions (exons) are linked together via the action of a ribonucleoprotein complex called the spliceosome. Spliceosome mutations are highly specific to MDSs and can be found in over half of all cases. They often may be the initial 'founder' mutation leading to the development of an MDS.

Therapy-related myelodysplastic syndrome

Approximately 15% of MDS cases are seen in those who have previously been exposed to either cytotoxic chemotherapy or radiotherapy (i.e. t-MDS). Alkylating agents (e.g. cyclophosphamide) and topoisomerase inhibitors (e.g. etoposide) are the common causative agents. t-MDS may also be seen as a late complication of haemopoietic stem cell transplant, due to proliferation pressure on the transplanted stem cells, altered micro-environmental interactions and direct genomic damage from chemotherapy and immunosuppressive agents. t-MDS usually presents 1–7 years after exposure to the implicated agent. As survivorship increases post-treatment of malignancies, an increase in the incidence of t-MDS will be observed, and close monitoring for any signs of development should be a key feature of any late-effects surveillance programme. Compared with other subtypes of MDS, there is a higher incidence of chromosomal abnormalities, such as loss (monosomy) of chromosomes 5 and 7, and a higher rate of progression to AML and a grim prognosis.

Presentation

An MDS should be suspected in any patient with unexpected cytopenia(s) or macrocytosis, as approximately 20% of those diagnosed with the condition will be diagnosed via an incidental finding of cytopenia(s) in bloods taken for unrelated reasons. Other potential presenting features of an MDS include fatigue (secondary to anaemia), bleeding (thrombocytopenia) and bacterial infections, such as skin abscesses or pneumonias (neutropenia). Otherwise, rare autoimmune conditions such as Sweet's syndrome and cutaneous vasculitis also have an association with MDS.

Investigation

A precise history and examination should be performed. A blood count and examination of a peripheral blood film can reveal characteristic features of dysplasia, but in order to make a definitive diagnosis a bone marrow aspirate and trephine is usually performed. As this is an invasive procedure it does not necessarily need to be performed in those who are asymptomatic and do not require intervention, as a watch and wait approach may be taken. Dysplastic features seen in the blood and marrow are summarised in Table 8.2 and Figures 8.1, 8.2, 8.3, 8.4 and 8.5. Cytogenetic analysis of either the peripheral blood or bone marrow sample is also essential for proper classification and prognostication of MDS.

When making a diagnosis of MDS, other causes of dysplasia or cytopenia should be considered and corrected. Differential causes of dysplastic features seen are listed in Table 8.3.

Classification

MDSs were previously categorised according to the French–American–British (FAB) guidelines, but these have been superseded by the World Health Organization (WHO) classification, summarised in Table 8.4. Major changes from the FAB classification include the removal of chronic myelomonocytic leukaemia (CMML) into a new category of myelodysplastic/myeloproliferative neoplasms, the reduction of blasts required to diagnose AML to 20% (previously 30%) and the creation of a new entity: MDS associated with isolated chromosome 5q – deletion. Specific examples are as follows.

Myelodysplastic syndrome associated with isolated 5q–

Predominantly seen in women, this category of MDS usually presents with symptomatic anaemia and thrombocytosis. The marrow examination shows increased numbers of dysplastic megakaryocytes, with relatively little dysplasia in the other cell lineages. The only cytogenetic abnormality is deletion of the long arm of chromosome 5. This subtype of MDS is associated with an excellent prognosis, and therapy has been revolutionised by the introduction of an immunomodulatory drug called lenalidomide.

Table 8.2 Dysplastic features.

Myeloid lineage	Blood film	Bone marrow
Erythroid	Macrocytosis	Multinucleate forms and nuclear budding
	Basophilic stippling	Cytoplasmic vacuolation Ring sideroblasts
Granulocytic	Nuclear hypolobulation (pseudo Pelger–Huët) Hypersegmentation Large cytoplasmic granules (pseudo Chediak–Higashi) Hypogranularity	As peripheral blood findings
Megakaryocytic	Hypogranular platelets	Micromegakaryocytes Monolobated nuclei Nuclear separation

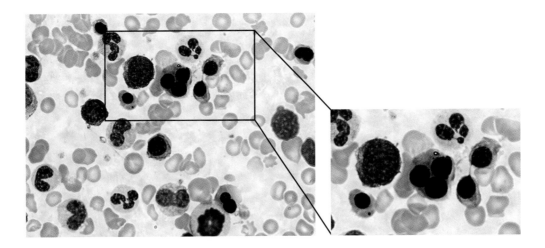

Figure 8.1

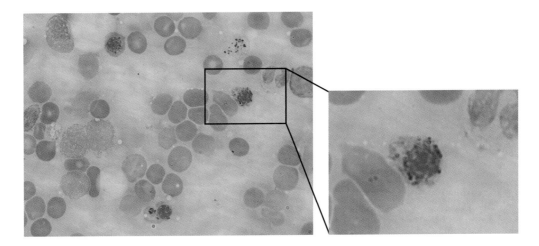

Figure 8.2

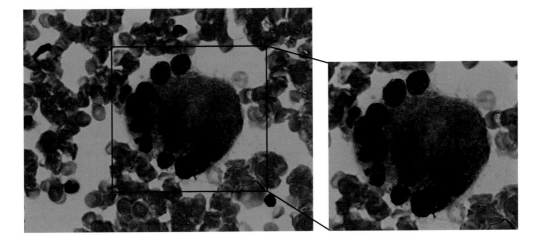

Figure 8.3

Myelodysplastic/myeloproliferative neoplasms

These are conditions that display features of both MDS and myeloproliferative neoplasms, the most common example of which is CMML. Defined by its persistent monocytosis, CMML is a challenging disease to treat with a highly variable prognosis (median survival 20–40 months) and a high rate of progression to AML (15–30% of cases).

Prognosis

As can be seen from Table 8.4, MDSs have a very varied prognosis, with survival ranging from months to years. This variation can make the therapeutic decision-making process more difficult. In order to give more accurate data about the prognosis the International Prognostic Scoring System (IPSS) was devised and published in

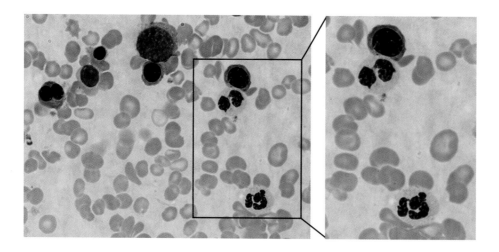

Figure 8.4

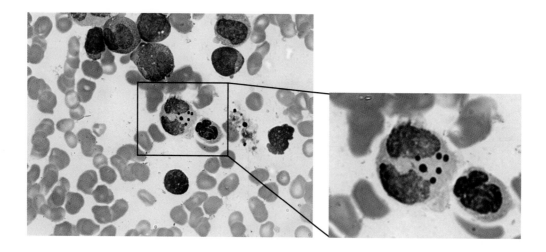

Figure 8.5

Table 8.3 Other causes of dysplasia.

Cause	Examples
Inherited	Congenital dyserythropoietic anaemias
	Congenital sideroblastic anaemia
	Thalassaemia
	Congenital dyserythropoietic porphyria
Severe systemic illness	Sepsis
Drugs	Co-trimoxazole
	Mycophenolate mofetil
Toxins	Excess alcohol
	Lead
	Benzene
Autoimmune diseases	
Micronutrient deficiency	B_{12} and folate deficiency
	Copper deficiency
Viruses	HIV
	Parvovirus
	HHV6

1997. Since then, a revision of the original scoring system has occurred to incorporate more up-to-date information about cytogenetic risks (R-IPSS). This new system predicts both overall survival and risk of transformation to AML (Tables 8.5 and 8.6). It

should be noted that the R-IPSS should only be used at diagnosis. If an estimation of prognosis is required at any other time a dynamic scoring system such as the WHO classification-based Prognostic Scoring System (WPSS) may be used (Tables 8.7 and 8.8).

Management

Owing to the variable nature of these syndromes, a stratified, individualised patient approach to management should be adopted, based on clinical and biological characteristics, disease subtype, patient choice and prognostic risk group. If possible, patients should be enrolled into clinical trials and entered into national registries in order to advance the understanding of MDSs and refine future treatment strategies.

Supportive care

Fundamental to the treatment of MDSs is the management of symptoms caused by cytopenias or reduced function of those cells. For those who are asymptomatic, a watch-and-wait approach may be most appropriate. In cases of symptomatic anaemia, red cell transfusions may be given, with a haemoglobin threshold determined on an individual basis. The use of the exogenous growth factor erythropoietin, administered subcutaneously, can

Table 8.4 WHO classification of MDSs.

Category	Cytopenias	Dysplasia	Blasts	Median survival (months)
MDS with single lineage dysplasia (MDS-SLD)	Unicytopaenia Bicytopaenia	Unilineage Multilineage	Blood <1% BM <5%	69
MDS with multilineage dysplasia (MDS-MLD)	Unicytopaenia Bicytopaenia Pancytopaenia	Multilineage	Blood <1% BM <5%	32
MDS with ring sideroblasts and single lineage dysplasia (MDS-RS-SLD)	Anaemia	Erythroid only >15% Ring sideroblasts or >5% if SF3B1 mutation	Blood <1% BM <5%	69
MDS with ring sideroblasts and multilineage dysplasia (MDS-RS-MLD)	Bicytopaenia Pancytopaenia	Multilineage >15% Ring sideroblasts or >5% if SF3B1 mutation	Blood <1% BM <5%	37
MDS with excess blasts-1 (MDS-EB-1)	Unicytopaenia Bicytopaenia Pancytopaenia	Unilineage Multilineage	Blood <5% BM 5–9%	18
MDS with excess blasts-2 (MDS-EB-2)	Unicytopaenia Bicytopaenia Pancytopaenia	Unilineage Multilineage	Blood 5–19% BM 10–19%	10
MDS with isolated del(5q)	Anaemia Normal or increased Platelets	Hypolobulated megakaryocytes	Blood <1% BM <5%	116

BM: bone Marrow.

Table 8.5 R-IPSS for MDSs.

	Score value						
	0	0.5	1	1.5	2	3	4
Cytogenetics	Very good		Good		Intermediate	Poor	Very poor
BM blast (%)	<2		≥2–<5		5–10	>10	
Haemoglobin (g/L)	≥100		80–<100	<80			
Platelets (×10⁹/L)	≥100	50–<100	<50				
Neutrophils (×10⁹/L)	≥0.8	<0.8					

Cytogenetics
Very good — −Y, del(11q)
Good — Normal, del(5q), del(12p), del(20q), double including del(5q)
Intermediate — Del(7q), +8, +19, i(17q) any other single or double independent clones
Poor — −7, inv(3)/t(3q), double including −7/del(7q), complex: 3 abnormalities
Very poor — Complex: >3 abnormalities

Table 8.6 Risk stratification for R-IPSS.

Risk score	Risk category	Median survival (years)	25% evolution to AML (years)
≤1.5	Very low	8.8	Not reached
>1.5–3	Low	5.3	10.8
>3–4.5	Intermediate	3.0	3.2
>4.5–6	High	1.6	1.4
>6	Very high	0.8	0.73

Table 8.7 WHO classification-based prognostic scoring system (WPSS).

	Score value			
	0	1	2	3
WHO Classification	MDS-SLD, MDS-RS-SLD ,5q–	MDS-MLD, MDS-RS-MLD	MDS-EB-1	MDS-EB-2
Cytogenetics	Good	Intermediate	Poor	
Transfusion requirement	None	Regularᵃ		

Cytogenetics:
Good — normal, −Y, del(5q−) only, del(20q−) only
Intermediate — all others
Poor — complex (≥3 abnormalities), or chromosome 7 abnormalities

ᵃ Defined as at least one red cell transfusion every 8 weeks over a period of 4 months.

Table 8.8 Risk category and prognosis.

Risk score	Risk category	Median survival (months)	Two-year probability of transformation to AML (%)
0	Very low	141	3
1	Low	66	6
2	Intermediate	48	21
3–4	High	26	38
5–6	Very high	9	80

benefit some patients with a reduction in transfusion requirements. Heavily transfused patients should be considered for iron chelation, in order to ameliorate the deleterious effects of iron loading in tissues such as the liver and heart. Febrile episodes in neutropenic patients are treated with broad-spectrum antibiotics and antifungals where indicated. The use of granulocytic colony stimulating factor, to stimulate granulocytic development, is often used in patients with neutropenia. Platelet transfusions can be used where there are bleeding symptoms or during intensive chemotherapy but are otherwise not recommended in stable thrombocytopenia. The use of thrombopoietin mimetics, such as eltrombopag, is not currently recommended outside of clinical trials as these increase bone marrow blast counts.

Immunomodulatory agents

The high incidence of autoimmune phenomena seen in MDSs provides some justification for the use of immunosuppressive agents such as anti-thymocyte globulin and ciclosporin or ciclosporin alone in those for whom transplant may not be a first-line option. Certain cytogenetic anomalies (e.g. trisomy 8) can predict response to immunosuppression.

Lenalidomide, an analogue of the immunomodulatory agent thalidomide, is licensed for use in those with 5q–MDS who are unresponsive to erythropoietin. Its use can reduce or abrogate transfusion requirements in up to 60% of patients.

Hypomethylating agents

Silencing of tumour suppressor genes via promoter hypermethylation has been implicated in the pathogenesis of MDSs. Hypomethylating drugs, such as azacitidine and decitabine, are well tolerated and can be administered in an outpatient setting. Azacitidine has been shown to increase overall survival by an average of 9.4 months and to reduce transfusion requirements when compared with both best supportive care and conventional chemotherapy. It is usually given subcutaneously, although trials of an oral formulation are underway.

Conventional chemotherapy

The use of low-dose cytarabine in MDSs has diminished but still has a role in certain individuals. Intensive, AML-type chemotherapy is used in selected patients to induce a remission prior to potential stem cell transplant.

Allogeneic stem cell transplantation

Stem cell transplant remains the only curative treatment for MDSs. Eligibility for transplant should be based on prognostic risk category, performance status, co-morbidities and patient preference. The use of reduced-intensity conditioning transplants means that patients previously considered unsuitable for transplant due to age can be given this treatment option. Fully human-leukocyte-antigen-matched siblings are the preferred source of stem cells, although unrelated matched donor transplants can have a similar outcome. Where no matched donor can be identified, alternative donor stem cell sources, such as umbilical cord blood or haploidentical donors, should be considered.

Future of the myelodysplastic syndromes

Advances in deep sequencing of both the genome and immune system will permit rapid evaluation of each individual for their specific mutation and immune profile. This will ultimately lead to refinements in disease classification and prognostication based on these findings. Furthermore, it will allow for therapies to be better targeted, either by predicting response to currently available therapies or by the use of novel treatments targeting specific dysregulated pathways.

Further reading

Boultwood J, Dolatshad H, Varanasi SS, Yip BH and Pellagatti A (2014) The role of splicing factor mutations in the pathogenesis of the myelodysplastic syndromes. *Advances in Biological Regulation*, **54**, 153–161.

Greenberg PL, Tuechler H, Schanz J et al. (2012) Revised international prognostic scoring system for myelodysplastic syndromes. *Blood*, **120**(12), 2454–2465.

Killick SB, Carter C, Culligan D et al. (2014) British Committee for Standards in Haematology, Guidelines for the diagnosis and management of adult myelodysplastic syndromes. *British Journal of Haematology*, **164**, 503–525.

Kohlmann A, Kuznia S, Nadarajah N et al. (2013) Diagnostic and prognostic utility of a 26-gene panel for deep-sequencing mutation analysis in myeloid malignancies. *Blood*, **122**(21), 1547.

Malcovati L, Germing U, Kuendgen A et al. (2007) Time-dependent prognostic scoring system for predicting survival and leukemic evolution in myelodysplastic syndromes. *Journal of Clinical Oncology*, **25**(23), 3503–3510.

Mufti GJ and Potter V (2012) Myelodysplastic syndromes: who and when in the course of disease to transplant. *Hematology, American Society of Hematology, Education Program*, **2012**(1): 49–55.

Schroeder MA and DeZern AE (2015) Do somatic mutations in de novo MDS predict for response to treatment? *Hematology, American Society of Hematology, Education Program*, **2015**(1): 317–328.

Swerdlow SH, Campo E, Harris NL et al. (eds) (2008) *WHO Classification of Tumours of Haematopoietic and Lymphoid Tissues*, 4th edition, IARC Press, Lyon.

CHAPTER 9

Multiple Myeloma

Sandra Hassan[1] and Jamie Cavenagh[2]

[1] Queen's Hospital, BHR NHS Trust, Romford, UK
[2] Department of Haemato-Oncology, St Bartholomew's Hospital, West Smithfield, London, UK

OVERVIEW

- Multiple myeloma is the second commonest haematological malignancy, with 4500 new cases per year in the UK.

- The commonest presenting features are bone lesions, hypercalcaemia, renal impairment and anaemia.

- Cytogenetic abnormalities have important prognostic implications.

- Over the last 10–15 years, 'novel agents' (e.g. bortezomib, thalidomide and lenalidomide) have been introduced into the treatment of myeloma.

- Outcomes for patients with multiple myeloma have improved more than in any other cancer over the last 10 years.

Epidemiology

Multiple myeloma accounts for 1% of all malignancies and 12% of all haematological malignancies. It has an overall incidence in the UK of 7.5/100 000 and is more prevalent in men. Over 70% of patients are over the age of 65 years when diagnosed, although 1% of patients are less than 40 at presentation. It is twice as common in Afro-Caribbeans, who are frequently diagnosed at a younger age than their Caucasian counterparts.

Pathogenesis

Myeloma results from a clonal proliferation of plasma cells derived from post-germinal centre terminally differentiated B cells. In all cases, myeloma is preceded by monoclonal gammopathy of undetermined significance (MGUS). Transformation of MGUS to myeloma occurs at a frequency of approximately 1% per annum. Multiple myeloma cells characteristically have cytogenetic abnormalities, most commonly hyperdiploidy and translocations involving the immunoglobulin (Ig) heavy chain gene (at 14q32). Additional cytogenetic changes, mutations and epigenetic abnormalities are also seen. These genetic abnormalities result in altered expression of adhesion molecules on plasma cells, allowing increased adherence to bone marrow stromal cells and haematopoietic cells. This results in the secretion of cytokines and growth factors such as interleukin-6 (IL6), vascular endothelial growth factor (VEGF), insulin-like growth factor and tumour necrosis factor-α. The complex autocrine and paracrine interactions between plasma cells and the bone marrow microenvironment result in tumour cell growth, angiogenesis and myeloma disease. Through activation of nuclear factor kappa B (NFκB), RANKL (receptor activator of NFκB ligand) is increased and the decoy receptor osteoprotegrin (OPG) is reduced resulting in increased osteoclastic activity. Plasma cells also secrete increased Dikkopf homologue 1 (DKK1) which inhibits the Wnt pathway. This in turn inhibits differentiation of osteoblast precursors. The resulting imbalance between osteoclast and osteoblast activity results in bone resorption and hypercalcaemia (Figure 9.1).

As the bone marrow is effaced with the clonal proliferation of plasma cells, normal haematopoiesis is suppressed, resulting in anaemia, and less commonly, other cytopenias.

Plasma cells secrete monoclonal antibodies which are responsible for clinical complications such as hyperviscosity (especially IgA) and renal failure as a result of light-chain deposition in renal tubules. The excess production of monoclonal antibody results in a depression in the production of normal Ig, leaving patients susceptible to infections, particularly bacterial.

Clinical features

In the early stages, myeloma may be asymptomatic and may be diagnosed as an incidental finding on blood tests done for another reason. However, myeloma may present with a variety of symptoms (Table 9.1, Figure 9.2). Many of the symptoms are non-specific, which often results in delayed diagnosis.

If myeloma presents with spinal cord compression (Figure 9.3), hypercalcaemia, renal failure or hyperviscosity, it represents a medical emergency and requires urgent investigation and treatment.

ABC of Clinical Haematology, Fourth Edition. Edited by Drew Provan.
© 2018 John Wiley & Sons Ltd. Published 2018 by John Wiley & Sons Ltd.

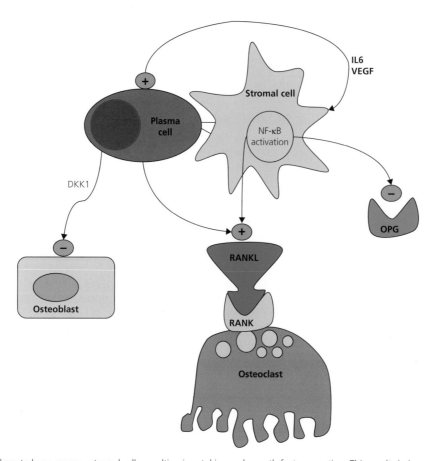

Figure 9.1 Plasma cells adhere to bone marrow stromal cells, resulting in cytokine and growth factor secretion. This results in increased osteoclastic activity and osteoblast inhibition, leading to bone resorption.

Table 9.1 Clinical features of multiple myeloma.

Symptom	Cause	Patients presenting with these symptoms
Bone pain	Lytic lesions Pathological fractures (Figure 9.2)	80–90%
Fatigue, shortness of breath	Anaemia	50%
Thirst, polyuria, nausea, constipation, confusion	Hypercalcaemia	30%
Nausea, loss of appetite	Renal failure	25%
Fatigue, appetite loss, weight loss	Cytokine release secondary to malignancy	25%
Recurrent infections	Hypogammaglobulinaemia, neutropenia	10% have fatal infections in first few months following diagnosis
Macroglossia, cardiac failure, peripheral oedema, peripheral neuropathy	Amyloid	10%
Headaches, blurred vision, mucosal bleeding, confusion	Hyperviscosity	2–6%
Back pain, leg weakness, sensory loss, incontinence	Spinal cord compression	5%
Bruising or bleeding	Thrombocytopenia	5%

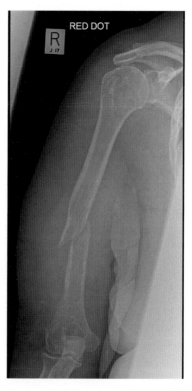

Figure 9.2 Radiograph showing pathological fracture of the humerus.

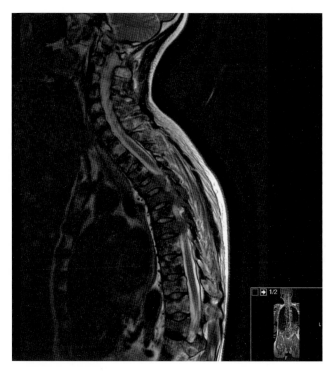

Figure 9.3 Magnetic resonance image showing compressive myelomatous infiltration at T4, T5 and T7.

Renal failure

There are several factors that may contribute to renal failure in myeloma:

- free light chains cause tubular damage (cast nephropathy)
- hypercalcaemia
- nephrotoxic drugs
- infection
- dehydration.

Diagnosis

The International Myeloma Working Group has established criteria for the diagnosis of myeloma and MGUS (Table 9.2).

The presence of any of the following 'CRAB' features allows the distinction between asymptomatic and symptomatic myeloma to be made. They must be ascertained to be directly attributable to myeloma in order for the diagnosis of symptomatic myeloma to be made.

- **H**yperCalcaemia
- **R**enal impairment
- **A**naemia
- **B**one lesions – lytic lesion (Figure 9.4) or osteoporosis with compression fractures
- Other – hyperviscosity, amyloidosis, more than two bacterial infections in 12 months.

There are several subtypes of myeloma, depending on the paraprotein detected:

- IgG (60%)
- IgA (20%)
- light-chain only multiple myeloma (kappa or lambda) (15%)

Table 9.2 Diagnostic criteria for multiple myeloma and MGUS.

Diagnosis	Diagnostic criteria	Presence of ROTI[a]
MGUS	Paraprotein ≤30 g/L and clonal plasma cells ≤10%	No
Asymptomatic myeloma	Serum paraprotein ≥30 g/L and/or clonal plasma cells ≥10%	No
Symptomatic myeloma	Paraprotein in serum or urine (no minimum level) (Approximately 1% have no detectable paraprotein – non-secretory myeloma) Clonal Plasma cells ≥10% or biopsy-proven plasmacytoma	Yes

[a] ROTI: (myeloma-)related organ or tissue impairment.

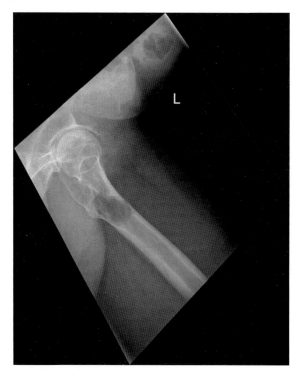

Figure 9.4 Radiograph showing large lytic lesion of the femur.

- IgD (2%)
- non-secretory (1%)
  - no detectable serum or urine paraprotein
  - 75% do have detectable serum-free light chains and invariably associated immunoparesis
- IgM (0.5%)
- IgE (0.01%).

The subtypes have different clinical phenotypes. Patients with IgA myeloma are at greater risk of hyperviscosity complications due to their large dimeric Ig structure. Some 50% of myeloma patients with renal failure have light-chain myeloma. The rare IgD, IgM and IgE subtypes are all associated with a worse prognosis. The presence of an IgM paraprotein is much more likely to be associated with the diagnosis of Waldenström macroglobulinaemia.

Investigations and staging

Investigations are performed to confirm the diagnosis, to establish the presence of end-organ damage and to evaluate prognosis.

Diagnosis
- Electrophoresis of serum and urine (Figure 9.5)
- Igs – if there is no detectable paraprotein but there is immunoparesis, this may suggest non-secretory myeloma
- Immunofixation of serum and urine
  - urinalysis is best done on a 24-h urine sample
- Serum-free light-chain assay
- Bone marrow aspirate and trephine (Figure 9.6).

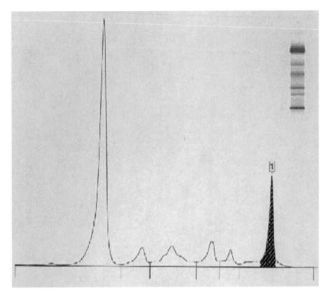

Figure 9.5 Protein electrophoresis strip showing IgG kappa serum paraprotein. The first and largest peak is albumin, which lies closest to the positive electrode. The next five peaks are alpha-1, alpha-2, beta-1, beta-2, and gamma. Within the gamma peak (shaded), a monoclonal IgG protein is characterised by the presence of a sharp, well-defined band.

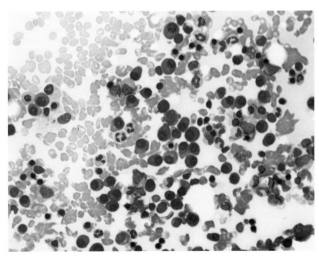

Figure 9.6 Bone marrow aspirate showing plasma cell infiltrate.

End-organ damage (ROTI) / other complications
- Full blood count.
- Serum urea and creatinine.
- Calcium.
- Skeletal survey.
- One of low dose whole-body CT, whole-body MRI or PETCT is recommended in all patients with suspected myeloma.
- Clotting profile (may be abnormal in the presence of amyloid which is associated with Factor X deficiency).
- Electrocardiogram/echocardiogram – to look for presence of cardiac amyloid, which may cause low-voltage electrocardiograms and concentric thickened ventricles.

Other investigations

If a patient has an IgM paraprotein, they should have a CT to look for lymphadenopathy or organomegaly suggestive of Waldenström's macroglobulinaemia (lymphoplasmacytic lymphoma).

If there is suggestion of amyloid light-chain amyloidosis, the patient should have a serum amyloid P scan to look for the presence of visceral amyloid. A tissue biopsy is required to confirm the diagnosis. The bone marrow trephine and any other tissue biopsies should be stained with Congo red to look for apple-green birefringence under polarised light.

Prognosis
- Albumin
- β_2 microglobulin
- Cytogenetic analysis by fluorescence in-situ hybridisation (FISH) on bone marrow.

The serum albumin and β_2 microglobulin concentration measured at diagnosis are used to calculate the International Staging Score (Table 9.3), which has now superseded the previously used Durie–Salmon staging system.

LOH and Cytogenetic profiles by FISH, whilst not formally incorporated into validated staging systems yet, are recognised to have prognostic value and may have an impact on therapeutic decisions.

The following chromosomal abnormalities confer poor prognosis:
- hypodiploidy
- t(4;14)
- t(14;16)
- 17p13 deletion
- amplification or gain of chromosome 1 (1q+ or 1p−).

Any chromosomal abnormality detected on metaphase cytogenetics confers a worse prognosis than a normal karyotype. The detection of t(11;14) confers standard risk disease.

Table 9.3 International Staging Score (ISS).

ISS	Albumin (g/L)	β_2 microglobulin (mg/L)	Median survival (months)
1	≥35	<3.5	62
2	Criteria fit neither 1 nor 3		45
3	Any value	≥5.5	29

Management

Myeloma is not a curable disease, and it is important that patients are made aware of this at diagnosis. The aim of treatment is to improve survival and quality of life. It is inevitable that, following treatment, even with prolonged responses, the disease will progress and treatment will be required again. Ultimately, a time will come when there are no further treatment options available or chemotherapy is no longer appropriate. The 10-year survival in patients under 60 is approximately 30%.

All patients should be managed by a multidisciplinary team with direct access to a clinical nurse specialist.

Patients with asymptomatic myeloma do not require treatment. However, they should be monitored regularly to look for progression to symptomatic myeloma.

All patients with symptomatic myeloma require treatment. They require myeloma-directed chemotherapy, but may also need additional supportive therapies (Table 9.4). The choice of initial chemotherapy depends on the age and performance status of the patient, and consequently on eligibility for autologous stem cell transplantation (ASCT).

Transplant-eligible patients

If the patient is ASCT eligible, the aim is to give a chemotherapy regimen that achieves a rapid response whilst being minimally toxic to allow the successful collection of stem cells following treatment. Myeloma therapy has been revolutionised over the last decade with the arrival of 'novel' agents. Indeed, survival for patients with myeloma has improved more than any other cancer over the last 10 years. This includes immunomodulatory agents such as thalidomide and lenalidomide and proteasome inhibitors such as bortezomib. All of these drugs form part of effective, well-tolerated induction regimens that can be used pre-ASCT. All can be given in the outpatient setting but all have potential toxicities, so patients

Table 9.4 Supportive treatment in myeloma.

Complication	Treatment
Lytic lesions/fractures	Bisphosphonates
	Surgical fixation/kyphoplasty
	Analgesia (no non-steroidal anti-inflammatory drugs due to risk of acute kidney injury)
	Radiotherapy
Renal failure	Intravenous hydration
	Dexamethasone and chemotherapy
	Dialysis
Hypercalcaemia	Hydration
	Bisphosphonates
Hyperviscosity	Plasma exchange
Cord compression	Dexamethasone
	Surgical stabilisation
	Radiotherapy
Anaemia and thrombocytopenia	Erythropoietin
	Blood and/or platelet transfusions
Infection	Prompt antibiotics
	Prophylactic antibiotics during treatment
	Annual influenza vaccine
	Ig infusion if recurrent infections

must be assessed regularly whilst on these treatments. Bortezomib- and thalidomide-containing regimens are the most commonly used in the UK with an over 80% response rate; for example, VTD (bortezomib, thalidomide and dexamethasone), CTD (cyclophosphamide, thalidomide and dexamethasone) and PAD (bortezomib, doxorubicin and dexamethasone). Most patients ≤65 years, who do not have significant co-morbidities, will undergo induction chemotherapy followed by an ASCT. This achieves a median overall survival (OS) of approximately 6–7 years. It is recognised that the achievement of a complete response (no detectable disease) is associated with improved progression-free survival (PFS) and OS.

Allogeneic stem cell transplant may be an option for selected patients and offers the prospect of cure offset by an increased procedure-related mortality.

Transplant-ineligible patients

In patients who are considered ineligible for ASCT, the aim is to give them treatment which achieves the best response with the least toxicity. As there is no concern about stem cell toxicity, they may receive alkylating agents such as melphalan in addition to novel agents. Regimens such as MPT/V (melphalan, prednisolone and thalidomide or bortezomib) are the standard of care in these patients offering a mean PFS of 1–2 years.

Treatment at progression

At progression, patients may receive the same agents again if they have been associated with prolonged responses previously. Alternatively, the patient may benefit from alternative therapies. They may also benefit from a second ASCT.

Future therapies

There are numerous clinical trials underway investigating the efficacy of oral proteasome inhibitors, newer immunomodulatory agents and monoclonal antibodies. As more effective therapies are identified, the question will be where they are best placed and whether ASCT will still be necessary.

Monoclonal gammopathy of undetermined significance

A detectable paraprotein <30 g/L with no evidence of end-organ damage is observed in 1% of the population. The prevalence increases with advancing age, and >5% of individuals >70 years have MGUS. The overall risk of progression to myeloma or other lymphoproliferative disorder is 1% per year, with a greater risk of transformation the higher the initial M protein is. All patients require monitoring, but those patients with IgG >15 g/L or IgA or IgM >10 g/L should be referred to a specialist.

Other plasma cell disorders

Other less common plasma cell disorders include solitary plasmacytoma of bone, extramedullary plasmacytoma and plasma cell leukaemia, which carries a much worse prognosis than multiple myeloma.

Further reading

Avet-Loiseau H, Attal M, Campion L *et al.* (2012) Long-term analysis of the IFM 99 trials for myeloma: cytogenetic abnormalities [t(4;14), del(17p), 1q gains] play a major role in defining long-term survival. *Journal of Clinical Oncology*, **30**, 1949–1952.

Ludwig H, Avet-Loiseau H, Blade J *et al.* (2012) European perspective on multiple myeloma treatment strategies: update following recent congresses. *Oncologist*, **17**, 592–606.

Palumbo A and Anderson K (2011) Multiple myeloma. *New England Journal of Medicine*, **364**, 1046–1060.

Pratt G, Jenner M, Owen R *et al.* (2014) Updates to the guidelines for the diagnosis and management of multiple myeloma. *British Journal of Haematology*, **167**(1), 131–133.

Stewart AK, Richardson PG and San-Miguel JF (2009) How I treat multiple myeloma in younger patients. *Blood*, **114**, 5436–5443.

CHAPTER 10

Bleeding Disorders, Thrombosis and Anticoagulation

David M. Keeling

Oxford University Hospitals, Oxford Haemophilia & Thrombosis Centre, Churchill Hospital, Oxford, UK

OVERVIEW

- Bleeding can be due to an inherited defect in platelets or coagulation factors.
- In a patient with bleeding, judicious use of screening tests and specialist coagulation tests can make the correct diagnosis and guide treatment.
- Haemophilia due to factor VIII or factor IX deficiency is an X-linked condition that can be treated with recombinant coagulation factors.
- Venous thromboembolism is due to venous stasis or hypercoagulability of the blood, sometimes due to a well-characterised inherited predisposition to thrombosis (a thrombophilia).
- Treatment of venous thromboembolism has for decades been with heparin and vitamin K antagonists (VKAs) such as warfarin but non-VKA oral anticoagulants are an alternative and do not require frequent monitoring and dose adjustment.

Blood within the circulation must remain fluid, but if a blood vessel is damaged, localised coagulation must take place to prevent loss of blood. When there is injury to a blood vessel, a series of events is initiated which results in controlled haemostasis. This involves:

- local vasoconstriction;
- adhesion and aggregation of platelets;
- activation of the clotting cascade, to form a fibrin clot;
- activation of coagulation inhibitors, to ensure coagulation is restricted to the site of injury;
- late fibrinolysis, to restore patency of the vessel.

These complex interacting systems can be disturbed by inherited or acquired factors, resulting in bleeding or thrombotic disorders.

Bleeding disorders

The approach to a patient with a suspected bleeding disorder involves medical history, examination, coagulation screening tests and specialist coagulation tests.

History and examination

When assessing a patient for a possible bleeding disorder, a good history is of paramount importance (Box 10.1). Is the bleeding mucocutaneous (Box 10.2) (often seen in platelet defects and von Willebrand disease (VWD)), or into joints and muscles (often seen in coagulation factor deficiencies)? The severity must be assessed. Did it result in anaemia or require a blood transfusion? These objective findings are important, as many normal people report that they 'bruise easily'. Particular attention must be paid to previous tests of the haemostatic system; for example, operations, dental extractions, trauma and childbirth. The age of onset and a family history are important to address the issue of whether the condition is likely to be inherited or acquired. Menorrhagia beginning from the menarche is much more likely to be due to an inherited coagulation defect than is menorrhagia starting later in life. If there is a family history, the mode of inheritance is important; for example, X-linked recessive inheritance suggests haemophilia A or B. Any other medical problems must be identified along with the use of any drugs which may affect haemostasis, such as aspirin or non-steroidal anti-inflammatory drugs. The common acquired causes of a coagulopathy, vitamin K deficiency, disseminated intravascular

---

Box 10.1 **History in a suspected bleeding disorder.**

- Type of bleeding: mucocutaneous, haemarthroses/muscle haematomas
- Severity of bleeding: blood transfusions, anaemia
- Previous tests of the haemostatic system:
  - operations
  - dental extractions
  - trauma
  - childbirth
- Age of onset
- Family history
- Other medical problems
- Drugs: aspirin, non-steroidal anti-inflammatory drugs

ABC of Clinical Haematology, Fourth Edition. Edited by Drew Provan.
© 2018 John Wiley & Sons Ltd. Published 2018 by John Wiley & Sons Ltd.

coagulation (DIC) and liver disease, must be considered, as well as conditions that may be mistaken for a coagulopathy (Box 10.3). The examination looks for evidence of bleeding and bruising but is mainly directed at detecting systemic disease.

Laboratory investigation

Most important coagulation disorders can be excluded if the pro-thrombin time (PT), activated partial thromboplastin time (APTT) and thrombin time (TT) or fibrinogen are normal. A full blood count will assess platelet numbers. Bleeding times are now rarely performed, but a platelet function analyser is sometimes used as a screening test for platelet defects. However, it is important to realise that mild VWD and some mild platelet defects, such as storage pool disease, can be missed by these screening tests, and if a bleeding disorder is strongly suspected then factor VIII, von Willebrand factor (VWF) activity and VWF antigen should be measured and platelet aggregation and platelet nucleotide measurements performed. If all these tests are normal in a case with a convincing history, deficiencies of factor XIII and α_2-antiplasmin should be considered (Box 10.4).

Figure 10.1 shows a simplified version of the coagulation cascade. This representation, although non-physiological, enables us to interpret the coagulation screening tests (Table 10.1). Heparin can sometimes prolong the APTT (and TT) without prolonging the PT, and occasionally a low fibrinogen may not be detected by the PT and APTT (hence the importance of either a TT or a direct measurement of fibrinogen).

Congenital bleeding disorders

Haemophilia A (factor VIII deficiency, with a frequency of 1 in 5000 male births) and haemophilia B (factor IX deficiency, 1 in 25 000 male births) are phenotypically identical X-linked recessive

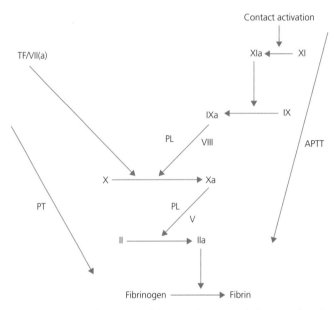

Figure 10.1 A simplified version of the coagulation cascade (TF: tissue factor).

Table 10.1 Interpretation of coagulation screening tests.

Result	Cause
PT prolonged, APTT normal	Deficiency of factor VII (seen in early vitamin K deficiency/oral anticoagulation or liver disease)
PT normal, APTT prolonged	Deficiency of factors VIII, IX, XI (or the contact factors)
	Lupus anticoagulant
PT prolonged, APTT prolonged, TT normal	Deficiencies of factors II, V, X
	Vitamin K deficiency/oral anticoagulation
	Liver disease
TT prolonged	Afibrinogenaemia
	Heparin
	DIC

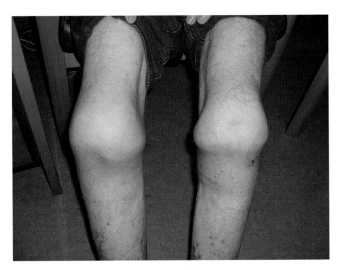

Figure 10.2 Knee arthropathy in haemophilia.

disorders. Patients with severe haemophilia (<1% factor VIII or IX) have spontaneous bleeding into muscles and joints that can lead to a crippling arthropathy (Figure 10.2). Patients with moderate (1–5%) and mild (>5%) factor levels usually bleed only after trauma or surgery. Management is usually undertaken in specialist haemophilia centres. Mild haemophilia A will respond to desmopressin, otherwise clotting factors are given. In developed countries, these are usually recombinant coagulation factors to avoid plasma-derived infections.

VWD is a common disorder caused by a reduction or structural abnormality of VWF. VWF has the dual role of promoting platelet adhesion to exposed collagen and protecting factor VIII in the circulation. In VWD, the main defect is the resulting abnormal platelet function and is manifest by mucocutaneous bleeding. Menorrhagia is common in affected women. Most cases are mild, with significant bleeding only occurring after a haemostatic challenge. Inheritance is usually autosomal dominant. Most patients with mild disease respond to desmopressin, but clotting factor concentrates are sometimes needed.

Acquired bleeding disorders

The common acquired coagulopathies are DIC, liver disease and vitamin K deficiency (Box 10.5). DIC occurs when a pathological stimulus to coagulation results in widespread microvascular thrombosis. This in turn results in a consumption of coagulation factors and platelets and a stimulation of fibrinolysis, which results in concurrent bleeding. It can be induced by conditions such as sepsis, trauma, malignancy, obstetric complications and severe transfusion

---

Box 10.5 **Common acquired coagulopathies.**

- DIC
- Liver disease
- Vitamin K deficiency

---

reactions. In liver disease, there may be loss of synthetic function, and, as the proteins of the coagulation cascade are synthesised in the liver, this can result in a coagulopathy often exacerbated by thrombocytopenia. An inadequate dietary intake or malabsorption of vitamin K will give a coagulopathy due to failure of γ-carboxylation of factors II, VII, IX and X.

Venous thromboembolism

Venous thromboembolism (VTE) – deep vein thrombosis (DVT) and pulmonary embolism (PE) – is due to a combination of blood stasis and hypercoagulability. The predisposing factors are shown in Box 10.6. In addition, a previous history of VTE is a strong risk factor, as this is a recurrent condition. Obesity, varicose veins and smoking are only weak risk factors.

Diagnosis is often made using a diagnostic algorithm which involves clinical examination (Figure 10.3), D-dimer (fibrin degradation fragment) testing and imaging investigations such as ultrasound. A typical diagnostic algorithm for DVT is shown in Figure 10.4.

Box 10.6 **Risk factors for VTE.**

- Age
- Immobilisation and paresis
- Surgery and trauma
- Malignancy
- Pregnancy and the puerperium
- The combined oral contraceptive pill
- Hormone replacement therapy
- The inherited thrombophilias
- Antiphospholipid antibodies
- Raised coagulation factors, e.g. factor VIII
- Family history of VTE
- Serious illness

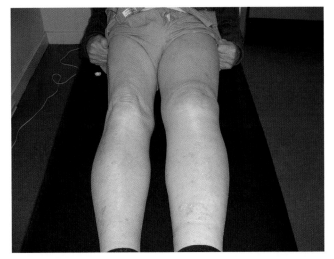

Figure 10.3 DVT.

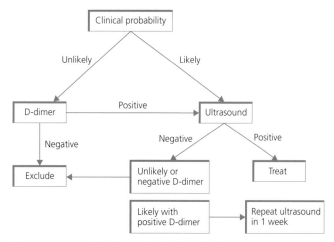

Figure 10.4 A possible diagnostic algorithm for diagnosis of DVT.

The inherited thrombophilias

The natural anticoagulant pathways are shown in Figure 10.5. Many of the coagulation proteins are serine proteases. Antithrombin is a member of a family of proteins known as serine protease inhibitors or serpins. It forms a one-to-one stoichiometric complex with serine proteases, thus neutralising them. As its name implies, its main effect is to neutralise thrombin, although it does also have significant inhibitory activity against factor Xa.

Activated protein C acts as a natural anticoagulant by cleaving the two cofactors in the coagulation pathway: factor V (FV) and factor VIII. To do this it needs its own cofactor, protein S. Proteins C and S are both vitamin-K-dependent proteins. The zymogen (inactive precursor form) protein C is activated by thrombin in the presence of an endothelial cell cofactor, thrombomodulin. It has been known for some time that deficiencies of antithrombin, protein C or protein S predispose to thrombosis. Heterozygotes for these deficiencies with 50% of normal levels are at risk, and therefore the thrombotic tendency is inherited in an autosomal dominant fashion.

Until 1993, these three deficiencies were the only well-characterised forms of inherited thrombophilia (Table 10.2). In 1993, the phenomenon of resistance to activated protein C was described. One year later, the molecular defect was identified as a G to A substitution at nucleotide position 1691 in FV. This results in the arginine at position 506 being replaced by a glutamine. Using the

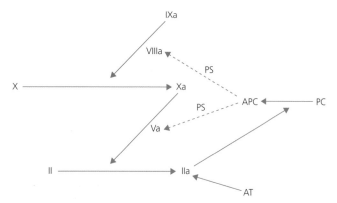

Figure 10.5 The natural anticoagulants. APC, activated protein C; AT, antithrombin; PC, protein C; PS, protein S.

Table 10.2 The heritable thrombophilias.

Condition	Prevalence
Antithrombin deficiency	1 in 3000
Protein C deficiency	1 in 300
Protein S deficiency	1 in 300
Factor V Leiden	1 in 20
Prothrombin G20210A	1 in 80

single-letter amino acid code, the mutant FV can therefore be written as FV R506Q, but is more often referred to as FV Leiden (Figure 10.6). Normally, FV is inactivated by an initial cleavage of the peptide bond at arginine 506, but the mutant FV is resistant to activated protein C. FV Leiden is present in 5% of the population, but is found in 20% of all cases of DVT, as it increases the risk of DVT approximately four- to sevenfold.

Shortly afterwards, it was discovered that a mutation in the 3′ untranslated region of the prothrombin gene, which is present in 1–2% of the population, is associated with an approximately three-fold increased risk of VTE. The mechanism is higher prothrombin levels in individuals with the mutation.

It is not recommended that all cases of VTE are investigated for inherited thrombophilia. To have utility the test result would have to change management. The National Institute for Health and Care Excellence (NICE) recommends that thrombophilia testing is not offered to patients who are continuing anticoagulation treatment but that testing is considered in patients who have had unprovoked DVT or PE and who have a first-degree relative who has had DVT or PE if it is planned to stop anticoagulation treatment (Box 10.7).

In addition to testing for inherited thrombophilia, consideration should also be given to testing for antiphospholipid antibodies, which are acquired and are associated with both venous and arterial disease. It is important to recognise that the inherited forms of thrombophilia are associated with venous thrombosis but not arterial disease.

Factor V Leiden (R506Q)

505	506	507
Arg	**Arg**	Gly
AGG	C**G**A	GGA
	↓	
AGG	C**A**A	GGA
Arg	**Gln**	Gly

Figure 10.6 The G → A point mutation results in the arginine at the protein C cleavage site being replaced by glutamine.

Box 10.7 **Considerations for testing for heritable thrombophilia.**

- Unprovoked or recurrent VTE plus
  - a first-degree relative who has had DVT or PE, and
  - it is planned to stop anticoagulation treatment
- Females of childbearing age who have a first-degree relative who has had DVT or PE and who has an identified heritable thrombophilia

Treatment of venous thromboembolism

Heparin

The initial treatment has historically been with heparin. Heparin is a mixture of glycosaminoglycan chains of varying length. Low molecular weight heparin, which has a mixture of shorter chains, has largely replaced unfractionated heparin. A specific pentasaccharide chain in the heparin chain binds to antithrombin and dramatically improves its ability to inhibit thrombin and factor Xa. The dose of low molecular weight heparin can be calculated by body weight and given subcutaneously once a day without any monitoring or dose adjustment.

Warfarin

Warfarin is a vitamin K antagonist (VKA), which prevents necessary post-translational modification of factors II, VII, IX and X. VKAs have been the mainstay of oral anticoagulation for decades, but alternatives now exist (see next subsection). Warfarin therapy is monitored by the international normalised ratio (INR; a manipulation of the PT to take account of the reagent used). For the treatment of VTE, the target INR is usually 2.5 (range 2.0–3.0).

Non-vitamin-K antagonist oral anticoagulants

Non-VKA oral anticoagulants which directly inhibit thrombin (dabigatran) or factor Xa (rivaroxaban, apixaban and edoxaban) are now available as an alternative to warfarin for stroke prevention in patients with atrial fibrillation and for treatment of acute VTE and long-term secondary prevention of recurrent VTE. They are not suitable for patients with mechanical heart valves. These drugs are given in fixed dose with no monitoring and no dose adjustment and therefore are more convenient to use than warfarin.

Further reading

Bates SM, Jaeschke R, Stevens SM *et al.* (2012) Diagnosis of DVT: antithrombotic therapy and prevention of thrombosis, 9th ed: American College of Chest Physicians evidence-based clinical practice guidelines. *Chest*, **141**, e351S–e418S.

Fijnvandraat K, Cnossen MH, Leebeek FWG and Peters M (2012) Diagnosis and management of haemophilia. *BMJ*, **344**, e2707.

Kearon C, Akl EA, Comerota AJ *et al.* (2012) Antithrombotic therapy for VTE disease: antithrombotic therapy and prevention of thrombosis, 9th ed: American College of Chest Physicians evidence-based clinical practice guidelines. *Chest*, **141**, e419S–e494S.

Keeling D, Baglin T, Tait C *et al.* (2011) Guidelines on oral anticoagulation with warfarin – fourth edition. *British Journal of Haematology*, **154**, 311–324.

Laffan MA, Lester W, O'Donnell JS *et al.* (2014) The diagnosis and management of von Willebrand disease: a United Kingdom Haemophilia Centre Doctors Organization guideline approved by the British Committee for Standards in Haematology. *British Journal of Haematology*, **167**(4), 453–465.

MacCallum P, Bowles L and Keeling D (2014) Diagnosis and management of heritable thrombophilias. *BMJ*, **349**, g4387.

CHAPTER 11

Lymphoproliferative Disorders

Catherine Hockings and Christopher McNamara

Department of Haematology, University College London Hospitals NHS Foundation Trust, London, UK

Introduction

Lymphoproliferative disorders (LPDs) are a heterogeneous group of conditions characterised by an abnormal proliferation of lymphocytes. The vast majority arise from mature B cells, but aberrations can arise at any stage of B or T cell maturation, leading to a diverse array of clinical conditions (Table 11.1).

Aetiology

Familial predisposition and geographical factors

Geographical factors can influence the epidemiology of LPDs. For example, Burkitt lymphoma is the most common childhood malignancy in equatorial Africa, but in western Europe comprises only 1–2% of lymphoid malignancies. This is thought to be induced by chronic malarial infection suppressing immunity to Epstein–Barr virus (EBV). T-cell lymphomas are more common in Asia, through a combination of racial predisposition and an increased seroprevalence of human T-cell lymphotropic virus type 1 infection. A higher incidence of human leucocyte antigen (HLA) haplotypes predisposing to gluten sensitivity in Welsh and Irish populations in turn leads to an increase in cases of enteropathy-associated T-cell lymphoma.

Immunosuppression

The incidence of B-cell neoplasms is markedly increased in patients with immunodeficiency. This may be inherited or acquired, as seen in human immunodeficiency virus infection. A specific EBV-driven LPD occurs in patients following marrow or solid-organ transplantation, referred to as post-transplant LPD. Reductions in patients' maintenance immunosuppression alone may be sufficient for disease regression in these cases.

Viruses

Viral infections are implicated in the pathogenesis of LPDs in both immunosuppressed and immunocompetent patients.

Table 11.1 WHO classification (major categories) of lymphoma.

Classification	Frequency of all lymphoma (%)	5-year survival (%)
Non Hodgkin's	60	
B lineage		
Diffuse large B-cell lymphoma	30.6	40
Follicular lymphoma	22.0	60
Marginal zone B-cell lymphoma/ mucosa-associated lymphoid tissue	7.6	70
Chronic lymphocytic leukaemia/ small lymphocytic lymphoma	6.7	>50
Mantle cell lymphoma	6.0	25
Primary mediastinal large B-cell lymphoma	2.4	70
Burkitt's/Burkitt-like lymphoma	2.5	85
T lineage	10	
Peripheral T-cell lymphoma	7.0	25
Anaplastic large cell lymphoma	2.4	70
Lymphoblastic lymphoma	1.7	30
Hodgkin's lymphoma (HL) (30% of lymphomas)	30	
Nodular lymphocyte-predominant HL	1.5	>90
Classical HL	28.5	>80
Nodular sclerosis classical HL		
Lymphocyte-rich classical HL		
Mixed cellularity classical HL		
Lymphocyte-depleted classical HL		

Chronic immune stimulation

Autoimmune conditions are associated with an increased incidence of LPDs. This may in part be due to inherited mutations in anti-apoptotic pathways, which both allow persistence of autoreactive lymphocytes and offer a survival advantage, with the acquisition of further somatic mutations leading to development of LPDs. Chronic inflammation of the salivary and thyroid glands is associated with increased incidence of marginal-zone lymphoma in Sjögren's and Hashimoto's thyroiditis respectively. Chronic stimulation of the immune system by bacteria can predispose to development of mucosa-associated lymphoid tissue (MALT) lymphoma at the site of infection, such as with *Helicobacter pylori* in the stomach.

ABC of Clinical Haematology, Fourth Edition. Edited by Drew Provan.

Presenting features

LPDs can present in a variety of ways, as discussed below.

Lymphadenopathy

Patients can present with either limited or widespread lymphadenopathy. This may be an incidental finding on imaging, or present as palpable lumps that have prompted the patient to seek medical attention.

Incidental lymphocytosis

Patients may present with an incidental finding of lymphocytosis on routine blood tests performed while monitoring another condition. More than 80% of chronic lymphocytic leukaemia patients are diagnosed in this way.

Autoimmune phenomena

Autoimmune disease can often occur as a paraneoplastic phenomenon; autoimmune haemolytic anaemia may be cold type, with monoclonal antibodies produced by the neoplastic clone, or warm type, with polyclonal autoantibodies resulting from immune dysregulation. Immune thrombocytopenia is also common.

Constitutional symptoms

"B" symptoms form part of the lymphoproliferative staging systems and are defined as fevers, night sweats (drenching, often prompting a change in nightwear or bedlinen) and weight loss (>10% of body weight in a 6-month period).

Extranodal disease and organomegaly

Advanced-stage disease can present with hepatosplenomegaly, often causing abdominal pain and swelling or early satiety. Organ dysfunction can also occur, either from extrinsic compression by lymph node masses or infiltration by extranodal disease.

Bone marrow infiltration

Replacement of normal haematopoietic tissue with disease in the bone marrow may result in fatigue and shortness of breath from anaemia, infections due to neutropenia or bleeding from resultant thrombocytopenia.

Hypercalcaemia

Heavy disease burden may lead to hypercalcaemia, with associated constipation, confusion and dehydration. In acute T-cell leukaemia/lymphoma (ATLL), expression of receptor activator of nuclear factor-κB (NF-κB) ligand induces differentiation of osteoclasts, resulting in hypercalcaemia in 50% of patients at presentation, often without concomitant osteolytic lesions.

Hyperviscosity

Although patients with chronic lymphocytic leukaemia (CLL) may present with an impressive absolute white cell count, symptoms of hyperviscosity, such as headache or visual disturbance, are rare, as the mature circulating cells are far smaller than the blasts or myeloid precursors of AML or CML. However,

prolymphocytic leukaemia (PLL), particularly T-cell PLL, consists of larger immature cells and may present in this manner.

Diagnosis

Blood film morphology

LPDs may present with a peripheral lymphocytosis (Figure 11.1). Microscopy can assist in identifying cells with an immature aggressive appearance, thus requiring urgent further investigations. Smaller differentiated cells suggest a more indolent mature entity. Blood film appearances can also guide appropriate panels for more definitive diagnosis with flow cytometry.

Flow cytometry

Flow cytometry can be performed on peripheral blood or bone marrow aspirate specimens. It provides immunophenotypic information at a single cell level, on thousands of cells – that is, far more than can practically be assessed by morphology. T- and B-cell LPDs have characteristic patterns of cell surface and cytoplasmic expression (see Tables 11.2 and 11.3).

Lymph node biopsy

Whole node excision biopsies provide helpful information about the disruption of normal lymph node architecture (Figure 11.2). However, inaccessible location of pathology (e.g. retroperitoneal nodes) and the relative ease with which image-guided biopsies can be scheduled mean that core biopsies are often presented to the haematopathologist. These provide some structural information, which can be supplemented with immunohistochemistry. Fine-needle aspiration is non-diagnostic and should be avoided. It is recommended that all LPD cases are centrally reviewed by an expert haematopathologist.

Bone marrow trephine

Sampling of bone marrow can provide diagnostic and staging information. The pattern of bone marrow involvement can also offer support for a diagnosis if characteristic; for example, paratrabecular involvement in FL.

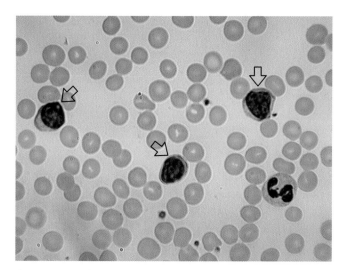

Figure 11.1 Peripheral blood smear of chronic lymphocytic leukaemia. Arrows = CLL cells.

Table 11.2 Flow cytometry expression patterns in common LPDs: B-cell neoplasms.

	CD20	CD23	CD5	CD10	sIG	CD22	CD79a	FMC7	Additional positives
CLL	+	+	+	−	+ (Weak)	+ (Weak)	+ (Weak)	−	CD200
Mantle cell	+	−	+	−	+ (Strong)	+ (Strong)	+	−/+	cyclinD1
Hairy cell	+	−	−	−	+ (Strong)	+	+	−/+	11c, 25,103,113
FL	+	−	−	+	+ (Strong)	+ (Strong)	+	+/−	Bcl-2, bcl-6,CD45, CD38
Burkitt's	+	−	−	+	+	+	+	+/−	HLA-DR, cCD79a, CD45
DLBCL	+	−	−	+/−	+ (Strong)	+	+	+/−	
B-PLL	+	−	−/+	−	+ (Strong)	+ (Strong)	+ (Strong)	−	
Marginal zone	+	−	−	−	+ (Strong)	+	+	+	11c

DLBCL: diffuse large B-cell lymphoma; FL: follicular lymphoma.

Table 11.3 Flow cytometry expression patterns in common LPDs: T-cell neoplasms.

	CD2	CD3	CD5	CD7	CD4	CD8	CD25	CD56
T-CLL	+	+	−/+	−/+	−	+	−	−
ATLL	+	+/−	+	+	+	−	+	−
Sezary	+	+/−	+	−/+	+	−	−	−
LGL	+	+	+	+	−	+	−	+
NK cell	+	+	−	+	−	+	−	+

LGL: large granular lymphocytic; NK: natural killer.

Gene expression profiling with microarray technology

Gene expression profiling (GEP) via microarray began as a research tool to identify therapeutic targets but is now on the cusp of being utilised for the initial diagnosis of LPDs.

Cytogenetics and molecular studies

Conventional karyotyping using G banding can be performed on fresh peripheral blood or bone marrow specimens. However, this may be challenging in low-grade LPDs due to the low proportion of cells in metaphase. Fluorescence in-situ hybridisation (FISH) can be used to target the characteristic translocations seen in many LPDs, often involving the immunoglobulin heavy chain gene (*IGH*) on chromosome 14 (see Table 11.4). The development of high-throughput parallel sequencing has led to the discovery of disease-specific mutations in LPDs, such as the *V600E BRAF* mutation in HCL and *L265P MYD88* in WM (Table 11.4).

Clonality studies

T-cell receptor rearrangement clonality can be established using techniques such as Southern blotting, PCR assays and now high-throughput sequencing.

Integrated reporting

The most accurate way to diagnose LPDs is by centralised integration of all of the aforementioned diagnostic modalities into a unified report. This should be internally validated and cross-checked, then distributed to the clinician treating the patient. Significant financial savings can be made via the omission of unnecessary tests, as well as avoiding the human cost of misdiagnosis.

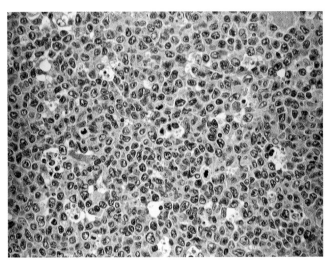

(a)

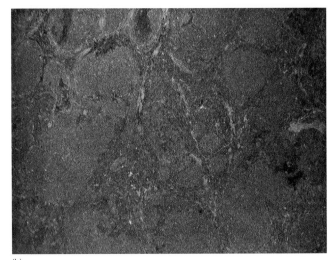

(b)

Figure 11.2 Lymph node microscopy (a) DLBCL-high power and (b) FL-low power note visible follicles.

Staging and prognosis

Once the diagnosis has been established, LPDs are staged in order to guide treatment strategies. This information will help tailor the optimal therapy for the individual patient. Staging systems used are the Ann Arbor for lymphomas (Table 11.5), largely incorporating imaging findings, and the Rai (Table 11.6) and Binet (Table 11.7) for CLL, which also include peripheral blood counts.

Table 11.4 Common genetic aberrations in lymphoproliferative conditions.

Lymphoma type	Mutation	Gene involved	Amount of mutation	Optimum testing method	Notes
FL	t(14;18)	IgH/Bcl2	~85%	PCR, FISH	Also in 15–20% DLBCL
HCL	V600F	BRAF	~100%	PCR/pyrosequencing	Also in 2.8% symptomatic myeloma
MCL	t(11;14)	CCND1/IgH	97%	FISH, PCR	Also in SMZL, CLL, B-PLL
WM	L265P	MYD88	79–100%	PCR	Also in 10% SMZL, 19% non-GC DLBCL, IgM-MGUS
Burkitt's	t(8;14)	c-myc/IgH	80%	FISH	Also in DLBCL
	t(8;2) or t(8;22)	c-myc/light chain locus	20%	FISH	
AITL/AL-PTCL	G17V	RHOA	~60% of each subtype	PCR	Not found in other haematological malignancies
CLL	17p deletion	TP53	Early disease: 5–7% Advanced refractory: 25–30%	FISH	Conveys poor prognosis and resistance to purine analogues
T-cell anaplastic	t(2;5)	ALK/NPM	~50%	FISH, RT-PCR	Conveys good prognosis

AITL: angioimmunoblastic T-cell lymphoma; AL-PTCL: AITL-like peripheral T-cell lymphoma; HCL: hairy cell lymphoma; IgM-MGUS: immunoglobulin M monoclonal gammopathy of undetermined significance; MCL: mantle cell lymphoma; non-GC: non-germinal centre; PCR: polymerase chain reaction; RT-PCR: reverse transcription PCR; SMZL: splenic marginal zone lymphoma; WM: Waldenström's macroglobulinaemia.

Table 11.5 Ann Arbor staging for lymphoma.

Stage	Criteria
I	Single lymph node region or single extralymphatic site
II	Two or more lymph node regions on the same side of the diaphragm; localized contiguous involvement of only one extralymphatic site and lymph node region (stage IIE)
III	Involvement of lymph node regions on both sides of the diaphragm; may include the spleen
IV	Disseminated involvement of one or more extralymphatic organs with or without lymph node involvement

Table 11.6 Rai staging of CLL.

Stage	Criteria
0	Lymphocytes >15 × 10⁹/L
1	Lymphadenopathy
2	Enlarged liver and/or spleen
3	Anaemia (haemoglobin <110 g/L)
4	Thrombocytopenia (platelets <100 × 10⁹/L)

Table 11.7 Binet staging for CLL.

Stage	Criteria
A	Lymphocytosis
B	≥3 areas of lympadenopathy[a]
C	Stage B + anaemia (haemoglobin <100 g/L)

[a] Lymph nodes areas: cervical, axillary, inguinal, hepatosplenomegaly.

Imaging

Computerised tomography (CT) has a long-established role in lymphoma staging. However, it provides anatomical information only. It has been complemented in some lymphoma subtypes by functional imaging with positron emission tomography using radionuclides with integrated CT to provide additional information regarding metabolic activity of tissues (see Figure 11.3).

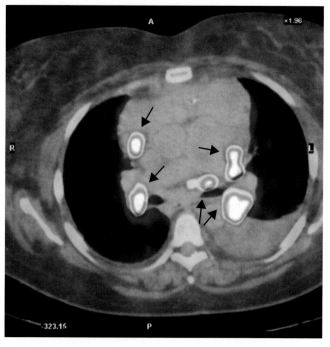

Figure 11.3 Interval CT/positron emission tomography scan showing residual metabolically active disease (arrows).

Bone marrow sampling

The incidence of bone marrow involvement varies greatly between lymphoma subtypes. Bone marrow aspirate and trephine biopsy are used to both stage disease and assess haematopoietic reserve in preparation for chemotherapy.

Prognostic scoring systems

Various clinical tools have been developed to aid clinicians in providing prognostic information to their patients. These incorporate staging and biochemical and haematological information, together with surrogate markers for the patient's ability to tolerate therapy, such as age or performance status (Tables 11.8 and 11.9).

Table 11.8 Lymphoma prognostic scoring systems.

Criteria	IPI	R-IPI	FLIPI	sMIPI
Age (years)	>60	>60	≥60	>50*
LDH	Raised	Raised	Raised	>0.67×ULN*
WHO performance status	≥2	≥3	—	≥2[a]
Ann Arbor staging	III/IV	III/IV	III/IV	—
Extranodal sites	≥2	≥2	—	—
Haemoglobin (g/L)	—	—	<120	—
No. of nodal areas involved	—	—	≥5	—
WBC count (/L)				>6.7×10⁹*

No. risk factors	3-year OS (%)	4-year PFS (%)	Median PFS (months)
0	Good, 91	Good, 94	Good, 84
1	Good	Good	Good
2	Low–Int, 81	Int, 80	Int, 70
3	High–Int, 65	Int	Poor, 42
4	Poor, 59	Poor, 53	Poor
5	Poor	Poor	Poor

LDH: lactate dehydrogenase; ULN: upper limit of normal; WBC: white blood cell; OS: overall survival; PFS: progression-free survival; Int: intermediate; IPI: international prognostic index; R-IPI: revised IPI; FLIPI: follicular lymphoma IPI; sMIPI: simplified MCL IPI (MIPI).
* Each criterion scored 0–3 based on degree of abnormality.

Table 11.9 European Organization for Research and Treatment of Cancer prognostic criteria for early stage Hodgkin's disease.

Favourable features	Unfavourable features
Age ≤50 years	Age >50 years
Nodular sclerosing or lymphocyte-rich histological variant	Mixed cellularity or lymphocyte-depleted histological variant
Stage I/II with <3 nodal involved areas	Stage II with >4 nodal involved areas
B symptoms with ESR <30 mm/h	B symptoms with ESR >30 mm/h
ESR <50 mm/h, absence of B symptoms	ESR >50 mm/h, absence of B symptoms
Mediastinal involvement <0.35 of thoracic diameter	Mediastinal involvement ≥0.35 of mediastinal diameter

ESR: erythrocyte sedimentation rate.

Other prognostic markers

Genetic or flow cytometric criteria can also be utilised for patients' risk stratification. In CLL, poor prognosis disease can be predicted biologically by unmutated immunoglobulin heavy chain genes. It's surrogate markers of ZAP-70 and CD38 positivity by flow cytometry are now in routine practice. Cytogenetic markers are also predictive of outcome in CLL, with p53 deletion being prognostic of poor response to fludarabine.

Treatment

As a general principle, high-grade disease is treated early with curative intent, whereas low-grade disease is treated only when resultant symptoms arise or vital organs are threatened, with a 'watch and wait' policy adopted in the interim. Other important considerations are the patient's fitness, co-morbidities, prognostic information and whether a clinical trial is available.

Conventional chemotherapy

The mainstay of treatment in advanced-stage disease is combination chemotherapy; for example, steroids plus alkylating agents, vinca alkyloids and anthracyclines. These regimens are generally delivered in cycles of 14–28 days, depending on the regimen and physician's choice.

Radiotherapy

Lymphoma is often highly radiosensitive. Relatively low doses of radiation are required for treatment compared with other solid tumours. Radiation fields, and therefore toxicity, are now much reduced compared with historical techniques.

Central nervous system prophylaxis and treatment

Risk assessment of patients with high-grade LPD should be carried out to establish the need for prophylaxis via intrathecal chemotherapy administration. High-risk patients can be identified by specific anatomical sites of involvement (testes, breast and epidural space) or a raised LDH with more than one extranodal site.

Monoclonal antibody therapy

The chimeric mouse/human monoclonal anti-CD20 antibody rituximab has been demonstrated to improve outcomes in almost every B-cell malignancy. It is included in upfront schedules for both high- and low-grade B-cell LPDs and has been approved for maintenance therapy in responders with FL.

Immunomodulatory therapy

As well as targeting clonal tumour cells, responses can be achieved by modification of their microenvironment. Lenalidomide has shown promising results in HL and lymphoplasmacytic lymphoma, acting to inhibit angiogenesis and modify cytokine signalling to tumour cells. Antibiotics alone are an effective treatment for gastric MALT lymphoma associated with *H. pylori* infection, inducing CR in up to 80% of patients without the need for more cytotoxic therapies.

Transplantation

Autologous and allogeneic transplantation are both widely used in the treatment of fit, chemosensitive patients with LPDs. In general, autologous transplantation is indicated in those patients achieving a complete remission to salvage chemotherapy, or after first-line therapy in those LPDs with a sufficiently high risk of relapse. Allogeneic transplantation, together with its additional complications and transplant-related mortality, may be used in refractory Hodgkin's disease, or with a reduced-intensity schedule in early relapse or high-grade transformation of low-grade LPDs in younger patients.

Small molecule B-cell signalling inhibitors

Next-generation sequencing and GEP projects have revealed upregulation of a variety of B-cell signalling pathways in many B-cell LPDs (see Figure 11.4). Pharmaceutical development of specific small molecule inhibitors has now reached clinical practice, with efficacy shown in various drugs with a variety of target pathways. Ibrutinib is an orally administered selective irreversible inhibitor of BTK. It has shown efficacy in a wide range of B-cell malignancies including hearing pre treated patients.

Supportive and holistic care

Much of the improvements in patient outcomes have come from improved supportive care. This includes infection control protocols, neutropenic dietary advice, against atypical infection prophylaxis and prompt antibiotic therapy in neutropenic sepsis.

Lymphoma subtypes

Classification

There are many subtypes of LPD, as detailed by the World Health Organization (WHO) classification system (Table 11.1). This takes into account morphology, protein expression by immunostaining, clinical features and signature genetic aberrations to characterise diseases. LPDs are broadly categorized into HL and non-HL (NHL), with the latter being further grouped into high- and low-grade and B- and T-cell disease. A brief overview of the features and treatment of the more common subtypes follows.

Hodgkin's lymphoma

HL was first described in the late 19th century with the discovery of tumours with giant multi-nucleate cells, the so-called Reed–Sternberg cells. These tumour cells in fact make up a minor component of the tumour bulk, with a reactive stroma of eosinophils, plasma cells and T-lymphocytes surrounding these large CD30 + ve cells (Figure 11.5). HL can be split into classical (95% of cases) and

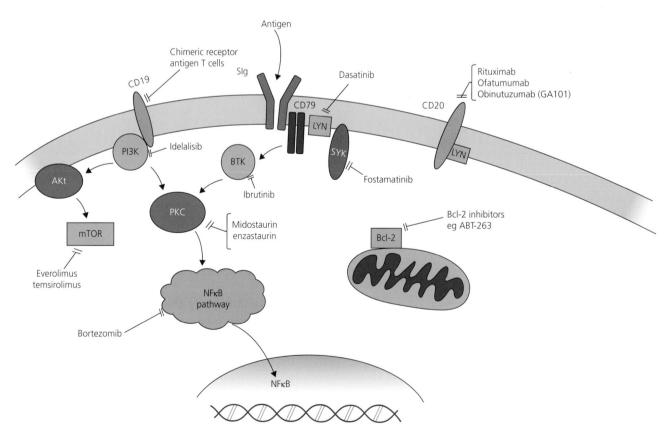

Figure 11.4 B-cell signalling pathways and targeted drug therapies. mTOR: mammalian target of rapamycin; NFκB: nuclear factor kappa-light-chain-enhancer of activated B cells; LYN: Lck/Yes novel tyrosine kinase (or tyrosine protein kinase LYN); PI3K: phosphatidylinositol 3-kinase; AKt: protein kinase B; PKC: protein kinase C; BCl-2: B-cell lymphoma 2; BTK: Bruton tyrosine kinase; SYK: spleen tyrosine kinase; SIg: surface immunoglobulin.

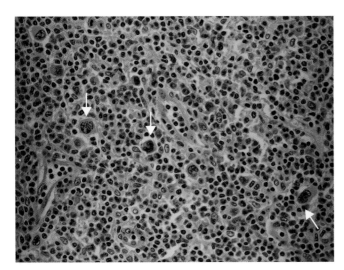

Figure 11.5 HL high-power view showing multiple large mononuclear Reed–Sternberg cells (arrows).

nodular lymphocyte predominant (5% of cases) subtypes, with the latter often being treated similarly to indolent NHL.

Diffuse large B-cell lymphoma

DLBCL is a high-grade NHL, which can arise *de novo* or as a transformation from indolent disease; for example, CLL (Richter's transformation) or FL. Two biologically distinct variants can be distinguished by immunohistochemistry or GEP. Germinal centre type has a superior outcome compared with the activated B cell subtype.

Follicular lymphoma

FL is a low-grade LPD, arising from germinal centre B cells. In affected nodes, the follicular pattern is at least partially preserved, but with absence of zonation (see Figure 11.2b). Cases are graded 1–3, according to the proportion of centroblasts observed. Grade 3B FL, defined by the presence of sheets of centroblasts, is treated similarly to DLBCL. FL cells express B-cell and germinal-centre immunohistochemical markers, as well as Bcl-2 due to the characteristic t(14;18) BCL-2; *IGH* translocation is found in approximately 85% of patients.

Burkitt's lymphoma

Burkitt's lymphoma is a B-cell NHL with an extremely high proliferation rate. Sporadic Burkitt's lymphoma is relatively rare and occurs throughout the world with a median age of onset of 30 years.

Patients often present with bulky disease and extranodal involvement. Immunohistochemistry shows a germinal centre B cell phenotype, with a characteristic *c-MYC* translocation detectable by FISH. This is partnered with *IGH* in 80% of cases t(8;14), with the other 20% displaying a light-chain variant translocation.

Chronic lymphocytic leukaemia / small lymphocytic lymphoma

The entities of CLL, monoclonal B-cell lymphocytosis and small lymphocytic lymphoma occur in a spectrum of clinical presentations. A diagnosis of CLL requires a monoclonal peripheral B-cell lymphocytosis of $>5 \times 10^9$/L for at least 3 months; small lymphocytic lymphoma requires the presence of lymphadenopathy without resultant cytopenias from bone marrow infiltration, with monoclonal B-cell lymphocytosis not meeting criteria for either but demonstrating B-cell clonality on flow cytometry.

The incidence of CLL increases with age, with a median age at diagnosis of 72 years in the UK. The Binet and Rai staging systems (see Tables 11.6 and 11.7) are predictive of outcome. Autoimmune cytopenias are common and are only an indication for cytoreductive therapy if they prove refractory to immunosuppression. Poor prognostic features such as p53 deletion should be investigated prior to treatment. FCR (fludarabine, cyclophosphamide, rituximab) is the most commonly used off-trial chemotherapy in the UK, in those patients deemed physically fit and without preclusive co-morbidities.

Mantle cell lymphoma

MCL is a B-cell LPD with features of both a high- and low-grade neoplasm. Patients often present with splenic and BM involvement, as well as other sites of extranodal disease, commonly the intestinal tract. There is a characteristic t(11;14) translocation involving cyclin D1, resulting in its overexpression and cell cycle dysregulation. The MIPI score has been established for MCL patients, with a proliferation index of >30% by Ki67 being an independent adverse prognostic factor.

Peripheral T-cell lymphomas

The mature T and NK lymphoproliferative neoplasms are a heterogeneous group of disorders, which can present as a lymphocytosis, nodal or extranodal disease, or with a cutaneous infiltration. They have a far lower incidence than the B-cell NHLs, comprising 10–12% of all lymphoid malignancies and, in general, have a poorer prognosis (5-year survival of approximately 30%). The most common subtypes in Europe are peripheral T-cell lymphoma not otherwise specified, anaplastic large cell lymphoma and AITL.

CHAPTER 12

Stem Cell Transplantation

Sandra Hassan[1] and John de Vos[2]

[1] Queen's Hospital, BHR NHS Trust, Romford, UK
[2] Royal Surrey County Hospital NHS Foundation Trust, Guildford, UK

OVERVIEW

- Most stem cell collections are obtained via peripheral blood stem cell harvest.
- Autologous stem cell transplant accounts for 60% of transplant activity. It is safe but results in frequent disease relapse.
- Allogeneic transplantation offers the only potential chance of cure in some haematological malignancies, but toxicities are much greater than autologous transplantation.
- The introduction of reduced-intensity conditioning has allowed allogeneic transplantation to be performed in older, less fit patients.
- The main toxicities of allogeneic transplantation are infection and graft-versus-host disease.

Introduction

Initially utilised as a treatment for those exposed to irradiation injuries, today stem cell transplantation offers the best chance of cure for many haematological malignancies. Transplant activity is increasing, with registered transplants in the UK approaching 4000 and 400 per annum for adults and paediatric practice respectively. Furthermore, its use has expanded to include not only non-haematological malignancies but also numerous non-malignant haematological and autoimmune disorders (Tables 12.1 and 12.2).

Stem cells

Stem cells are found within the bone marrow and are a self-renewing population of cells that are able to restore normal haematopoiesis. The aim of stem cell transplantation is to transfuse healthy stem cells into a patient after their bone marrow producing abnormal cells has been treated with chemotherapy.

Stem cell collection

Stem cells may be collected via bone marrow harvest or peripheral blood stem cell (PBSC) harvest. Today, the majority of paediatric stem cell collections are bone marrow harvests,

Table 12.1 Use of stem cell transplantation in adult practice (in order of frequency)

Autologous transplantation
  Multiple myeloma
  Non-Hodgkin lymphoma
  Hodgkin lymphoma
  Autoimmune disorders, e.g. multiple sclerosis, rheumatoid arthritis
  Neuroblastoma and germ-cell tumours
  Acute myeloid leukaemia
Allogeneic transplantation
  Acute myeloid leukaemia in CR1
  Myelodysplasia
  Relapsed acute myeloid leukaemia
  Relapsed non-Hodgkin lymphoma
  Acute lymphoblastic leukaemia in CR1
  Chronic lymphocytic leukaemia
  Myeloproliferative syndromes
  Bone marrow failure syndromes
  Chronic myeloid leukaemia in chronic phase
  Chronic myeloid leukaemia not in chronic phase
  Relapsed acute lymphoblastic leukaemia in CR1
  Hodgkin lymphoma
  Multiple myeloma

CR1: first complete remission.

whereas most adult stem cell donations are obtained via peripheral blood.

Bone marrow harvesting involves the donor receiving a general anaesthetic and 600–1200 mL bone marrow being aspirated from the iliac crests. Complications are those associated with receipt of a general anaesthetic and pain at the site following the procedure. PBSCs are obtained by administering haematopoietic growth factors to the donor which increase the number of circulating PBSCs. Stem cells can be identified by expression of CD34, a cell surface glycoprotein, and can therefore be separated from other circulating cells based upon their CD34 expression. Growth factor injections can result in bone pain, but there is no evidence to support an increased risk of haematological malignancy.

ABC of Clinical Haematology, Fourth Edition. Edited by Drew Provan.
© 2018 John Wiley & Sons Ltd. Published 2018 by John Wiley & Sons Ltd.

Table 12.2 Use of stem cell transplantation in paediatric practice (in order of frequency).

Autologous transplant
   Solid tumours, e.g. germ cell and neuroblastoma
   Hodgkin lymphoma
   Non-Hodgkin lymphoma
Allogeneic transplant
   Primary immunodeficiencies
   Bone marrow aplasias
   Relapsed acute lymphoblastic leukaemia
   Relapsed acute myeloid leukaemia
   Other inherited disorders
   Haemoglobinopathies
   Acute lymphoblastic leukaemia in CR1
   Myelodysplasia
   Histiocytic disorders
   Acute myeloid leukaemia in CR1
   Chronic myeloid leukaemia in chronic phase
   Non-Hodgkin lymphoma
   Hodgkin lymphoma
   Chronic myeloid leukaemia not in chronic phase

Autologous stem cell transplantation

There are different types of stem cell transplantation, as listed in Table 12.3. Autologous stem cell transplantation involves administration of high-dose chemotherapy followed by reinfusion of stem cells, previously harvested from the same patient. It is the most common type of transplant procedure, accounting for approximately 60% of adult transplant practice in the UK. It is performed most commonly for patients with multiple myeloma and relapsed lymphoma. Other uses are listed in Tables 12.1 and 12.2.

In myeloma, standard conditioning is with melphalan 200 mg/m². Autologous transplantation is used mostly in first response and is recognised to increase both progression-free survival and overall survival. Transplant-related mortality is low at 2–3%, but it is not a curative procedure in this setting. Toxicity includes a 2–3-week neutropenic period with mucositis and infectious complications.

In relapsed non-Hodgkin and Hodgkin lymphoma, autologous transplantation is considered standard of care if the patient is considered fit enough for the procedure and demonstrates chemosensitivity prior to transplantation. Standard conditioning in this setting is carmustine, etoposide, cytarabine and melphalan.

The greatest challenge in autologous transplantation is contamination of the collected stem cells by malignant cells, resulting in relapse for many. Attempts to purge the stem cell collection have

Table 12.3 Types of stem cell transplant.

Autologous (stem cells previously harvested from same patient)
Syngeneic (stem cells from identical twin)
Allogeneic
   HLA-matched sibling
   HLA-matched family member
   HLA-matched unrelated donor
   HLA-mismatched unrelated donor
   Haploidentical sibling/unrelated donor
   Umbilical cord blood donor

HLA: human leucocyte antigen.

not demonstrated any benefit. Other late complications may include infertility and increased risk of secondary malignancy.

Allogeneic stem cell transplantation

Allogeneic stem cell transplantation utilises myeloablative or reduced-intensity conditioning followed by the infusion of stem cells from a sibling or unrelated donor in most cases. Immunosuppressive drugs such as ciclosporin and methotrexate are usually given for a period of months post-transplant to suppress the 'host versus graft' effect and reduce the chances of graft rejection. Myeloablative conditioning is comprised of cyclophosphamide and total body irradiation or busulphan and cyclophosphamide. Transplant-related mortality is high, secondary to organ toxicity, graft-versus-host disease (GvHD) and infection, limiting its use to young, fit patients.

In the late 1970s, the graft-versus-leukaemia (GvL) effect was reported, supported by the following observations:

* concurrent achievement of remission following a graft-versus-host reaction;
* the occurrence of GVHD being associated with a reduction in disease relapse;
* the use of immunosuppression withdrawal and donor lymphocyte infusion to achieve remission in those who had relapsed post-transplant.

The understanding of the immunological processes involved in allogeneic transplantation resulted in the introduction of reduced-intensity conditioning in the late 1990s. This carried significantly less toxicity and increased the age range and performance status of patients that could undergo a stem cell transplant. However, the transplant-related mortality in allogeneic transplantation is still high, ranging between 10% and 40% depending on the disease, status at transplant and conditioning.

Donor selection

The identification of the most suitable donor is based upon HLA typing and matching of the recipient and potential donors. The HLA genes are carried on chromosome 6 and inherited as haplotypes, which means that a sibling has a 1:4 chance of being a match. If a patient does not have a matched sibling, a search for an unrelated donor will be carried out. There are national and international donor registries with over 23 million donors now available worldwide, and approximately 50% of patients will have an identified donor. Those from ethnic minorities have the lowest chance because the ethnic make-up of the largest donor registries remains largely Caucasian. All potential donors must be medically assessed to be fit to donate stem cells.

Consideration may be given to utilising an alternative donor. These include umbilical cord donors and haploidentical donors. Potential complications are higher using these stem cell sources but may be the best option in the absence of a fully matched donor.

Other factors considered in donor selection are donor age, gender, blood group and cytomegalovirus (CMV) antigen status.

Complications of allogeneic stem cell transplantation

The morbidity and mortality associated with this treatment remains significant despite ongoing refinements. The two largest causes of mortality are infectious complications and GvHD. Other toxicities are listed in Table 12.4.

Infection

Patients will receive prophylactic antibiotics, antivirals and antifungal medications during and after the transplant. Patients are also at risk of *Pneumocystis jiroveci*, and therefore receive co-trimoxazole as prophylaxis from engraftment.

The nature of the infective pathogens likely to occur is dependent on the time post-transplant. Early complications in the neutropenic period prior to engraftment include bacterial Gram-positive and Gram-negative, viral and fungal infections with *Candida* species and invasive *Aspergillus fumigatus*. Community respiratory viral pathogens such as respiratory syncytial virus, influenza and parainfluenza may be associated with significant risk of pneumonitis and secondary infection at early and intermediate stages post-transplant.

Following engraftment, and for several months post-transplant, patients are at risk of CMV reactivation, which occurs in 40–80% of at-risk individuals. CMV reactivation may progress to CMV disease, including pneumonitis, gastrointestinal ulceration, hepatitis and retinitis. CMV disease was previously the commonest cause of infectious death post-transplantation. Now, however, sensitive diagnostic tests may detect early viral reactivation in the blood and allow pre-emptive therapy with antiviral drugs. This has reduced both the occurrence of CMV disease and associated mortality.

Herpes zoster reactivation is seen in 40% of at-risk patients and may disseminate and rarely cause systemic and neurological infection.

Patients are advised to receive life-long penicillin V as prophylaxis against encapsulated organisms, particularly following ablative regimens. At 3 months post-transplant, it is recommended that patients undergo complete revaccination of childhood immunisations. However, they must not receive any live vaccines due to impaired cellular immunity and risk of infection until at least 2 years post-transplant with no evidence of GvHD and no ongoing immunosuppressive therapy. Late infectious deaths are seen particularly in patients with chronic GvHD (cGvHD) requiring immune suppression.

Graft-versus-host disease

GvHD is an immune response with organ injury mediated by donor T cells and inflammatory cytokines. It is traditionally divided into acute GvHD (aGvHD) and cGvHD (Table 12.5). It is responsible for significant morbidity and mortality post-transplant. The introduction of PBSC harvest resulted in more rapid engraftment, but the increased number of T cells in peripheral blood also resulted in increased cGvHD. Strategies to reduce GvHD include the administration of cyclosporine and methotrexate post-transplant and T-cell depletion of the graft. Whilst highly effective at reducing the risk of severe aGvHD, intensive T-cell depletion does significantly affect immune reconstitution and, importantly, increases the risk of disease relapse by also removing donor T cells that may mount a GvL response. Trying to delineate the GvL effect from GvHD is the subject of active research.

Acute graft-versus-host disease

aGvHD was historically defined as occurring within the first 100 days post-transplant. However, it is now recognised that GvHD that is clinically characteristic of aGvHD may occur beyond this time point, particularly following withdrawal of immune suppression (late-onset aGvHD).

Characteristic presentations include a skin rash, deranged liver function tests and diarrhoea. The skin is the most commonly affected site. The rash is typically an erythematous macular–papular rash that classically starts on the palms and soles but may spread to all sites (Figure 12.1). In its most severe form, there may be extensive erythroderma and bullae formation with mucocutaneous involvement.

Liver GvHD classically presents with a cholestatic liver picture with rising bilirubin and alkaline phosphatase. The differential of abnormal liver function tests post-transplant is wide, particularly if it occurs in the absence of GvHD affecting other organs. Liver biopsy may be useful, although practically difficult, if there is associated thrombocytopenia or coagulopathy. Characteristic histology demonstrates lymphocytic infiltration of the portal areas, pericholangitis and bile-duct loss.

aGvHD of the gut most commonly presents with secretory diarrhoea. Abdominal pain, nausea, vomiting, anorexia, weight loss, bleeding from ulcerated sites and ileus may also occur. Biopsies

Table 12.4 Complications post-transplant.

Acute	Chronic
Cytopenias and need for blood products	Chronic GvHD
Hair loss	Effects of prolonged corticosteroid use
Nausea and vomiting	Hypogammaglobulinaemia
Mucositis	Late infections
Sinusoidal obstruction syndrome	Infertility
Transplant-related lung injury	Hypothyroidism
Infection	Sexual dysfunction
bacterial	Cataracts
viral (e.g. CMV reactivation)	Depression and anxiety
fungal	Secondary malignancies
GvHD	

Table 12.5 Definitions of aGvHD and cGvHD.

	Timing	Presence of acute features	Presence of chronic features
aGvHD			
Classic acute	≤100 days	Yes	No
Persistent, recurrent, or late-onset acute	>100 days	Yes	No
cGvHD			
Classic chronic	No time limit	No	No
Overlap syndrome	No time limit	Yes	Yes

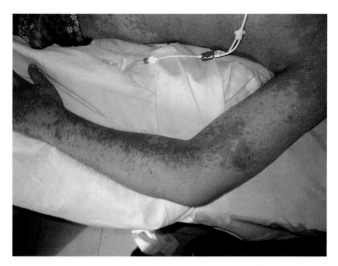

Figure 12.1 Skin involvement in GvHD.

taken at endoscopy may show patchy ulceration, apoptotic bodies at crypt bases, crypt ulceration and flattening of surface epithelium.

Biopsies may be helpful, but should not delay initiation of treatment. aGvHD should be graded according to the modified Seattle–Glucksberg criteria. Mortality of those with grade IV

aGvHD is over 90%. Isolated cutaneous GvHD may be managed with topical steroid creams. Patients with grade II–IV disease are likely to require systemic immunosuppression. First-line treatment is with high-dose corticosteroids. Second-line immunosuppressive drugs may be required. Non-absorbable steroids, such as budesonide, are useful in gut and liver aGvHD.

Chronic graft-versus-host disease

cGvHD is the most common late complication of long-term survivors of allogeneic stem cell transplantation and the leading cause of non-relapse mortality. It is reported to occur in 25–60% of patients. It was historically defined as occurring more than 100 days post-transplant but it is now recognised that classical features of cGvHD may occur within 100 days and may also occur concurrently with aGvHD. Consequently, there are now two subcategories for cGvHD: 'classic' and 'overlap' syndrome. It is a complex, often multisystem, disorder and is characterised by 'diagnostic' and 'distinctive' features (Table 12.6). The grading of cGvHD differs from that of aGvHD and can be graded as mild, moderate or severe according to National Institutes of Health consensus criteria.

Patients with extensive cGvHD often require long-term immunosuppressive therapy. First-line treatment is with corticosteroids, but the use of second-line immunosuppressive agents is

Table 12.6 Clinical characteristics of cGvHD.

Organ	Diagnostic[a]	Distinctive[b]
Skin	Poikiloderma Lichen planus-like features Morphea-like features Lichen sclerosus-like features	Depigmentation
Gastrointestinal	Oesophageal web Strictures or stenosis in the upper to mid third of the oesophagus	
Mouth	Lichen-type features Hyperkeratotic plaques Restriction of mouth opening from sclerosis	Xerostomia
Lung	Bronchiolitis obliterans diagnosed with lung biopsy	Bronchiolitis obliterans diagnosed with pulmonary function tests and radiology
Muscles, fascia, joints	Fasciitis Joint stiffness or contractures secondary to sclerosis	Myositis or polymyositis
Nails		Dystrophy Longitudinal ridging, splitting, brittle features Onycholysis Pterygium unguis Nail loss
Scalp and body hair		New onset of scarring/non-scarring scalp alopecia Scaling, papulosquamous lesions Mucocele Mucosal atrophy Pseudomembranes, ulcers
Eyes		New-onset dry, gritty or painful eyes Cicatricial conjunctivitis Keratoconjunctivitis sicca Confluent areas of punctate keratopathy

[a] Sufficient to establish the diagnosis of cGvHD.
[b] Insufficient alone to establish a diagnosis of cGvHD.

frequent, and extracorporeal photophoresis as a useful alternative treatment strategy. Infectious complications due to complex immune deficiency are frequent in this cohort and are the major cause of death.

Conclusions

Stem cell transplantation is continuously evolving, and the introduction of reduced-intensity conditioning has opened up this treatment strategy to a much wider cohort of patients. However, two fundamental problems remain: first, the associated toxicities; and second, the significant rate of relapse that still occurs post-transplant. Novel therapeutic agents, including molecularly targeted drugs, immunomodulatory agents and gene therapies, are changing the scene in the treatment of haematological malignancies and attempting to challenge the role of transplantation. Research is ongoing, aiming to delineate the immune mechanisms involved in the the GvL and GvHD processes in addition to improving disease-stratification, vaccination therapy, adoptive immunotherapy and the use of post-transplant maintenance therapy. The aspiration is that stem cell transplantation can one day become a highly refined treatment with minimal toxicity and high cure rates.

Further reading

Ljungman P, Bregni M, Brune M *et al.* (2010) Allogeneic and autologous transplantation for haematological diseases, solid tumours and immune disorders: current practice in Europe 2009. *Bone Marrow Transplantation*, **45**, 219–234.

McSweeney P, Niederwieser D, Shizuru J *et al.* (2001) Hematopoietic cell transplantation in older patients with hematologic malignancies: replacing high-dose cytotoxic therapy with graft-versus-tumor effects. *Blood*, **97**(11), 3390–3400.

Gratwohl A, Brand R, Frassoni F *et al.* (2005) Cause of death after allogeneic haematopoietic stem cell transplantation (HSCT) in early leukaemias: an EBMT analysis of lethal infectious complications and changes over calendar time. *Bone Marrow Transplantation*, **36**, 757–769.

Filipovich A (2008) Diagnosis and manifestations of chronic graft-versus-host disease. *Best Practice & Research Clinical Haematology*, **21**(2), 251–257.

Reisner Y, Aversa F and Martelli M (2015) Haploidentical hematopoietic stem cell transplantation: state of art. *Bone Marrow Transplantation*, **50**, S1–S5.

CHAPTER 13

Haematological Problems in Older Adults

Tom Butler[1] and Adrian C. Newland[1,2]

[1] Department of Clinical Haematology, Barts Health NHS Trust, Royal London Hospital, London, UK
[2] Barts and the London Medical School, Queen Mary University of London, London, UK

OVERVIEW

- The number of older patients is increasing worldwide.
- Challenges exist in defining anaemia in older adults.
- Anaemia is associated with morbidity and mortality in older adults.
- The cause of anaemia is often multifactorial.
- Haematological malignancies increase in incidence as people age.

Introduction

The global population proportion of older people (aged 60 years or over) increased from 9.2% in 1990 to 11.7% in 2013 and will continue to grow as a proportion of the world population, reaching 21.1% by 2050 (www.who.int/ageing). Globally, the number of older adults is expected to more than double, from 841 million people in 2013 to more than 2 billion in 2050. Older persons are projected to exceed the number of children for the first time in 2047.

Anaemia

Defining the normal ranges for haematological parameters is dependent on many factors, including age. To determine the normal range for haemoglobin (Hb), a healthy population is identified and the convention is to define the normal range by 95% confidence intervals. Defining a normal range in older adults poses challenges. Identifying a healthy older adult population is difficult due to the high incidence of disease, with often multiple morbidities. Extrapolating a definition of normal based on healthy younger adults to an older group may not be practically useful.

The conventional World Health Organization definition of anaemia is generally accepted, but the original studies did not include people >65 years of age:

- Hb <130 g/L for men
- Hb <120 g/L for women.

Defining anaemia by setting a lower limit of Hb is not equivalent to stating that a particular level is at an optimal value. There is some

evidence that higher 'normal' Hb values may be beneficial in older adults. Morbidity and mortality are lowest with Hb in the range 140–150 g/L, all-cause mortality increasing with higher or lower values. Some have called for abandoning a lower limit to define anaemia as 'low normal' Hb may be associated with morbidity, and underlying conditions may be missed. Importantly, studies have not been designed to assess causality; that is, whether morbidity is due to anaemia itself or the underlying cause of the anaemia.

There is a correlation between lower Hb levels and decreased physical or mental function and increased mortality. However, mortality also depends on the cause of the anaemia, with anaemia due to renal impairment associated with a higher mortality compared with anaemia due to nutritional deficiency.

Owing to variability in the populations studied or definitions of anaemia and older adulthood, the reported prevalence varies according to the study performed. The incidence increases with age, and there is a high rate in institutionalised people, particularly in hospital inpatients:

- >65 years 10%
- >85 years 20–25%
- >65 years, in hospital, 40–50%.

In general, anaemia in older adults is mild, with 10% of older anaemic patients classified as having 'severe' anaemia with an Hb <100 g/L.

The causes of anaemia in the older adult were evaluated in a study of a non-institutionalised US population in the third National Health and Nutrition Examination Survey. Amongst other things, this study looked at the causes of anaemia in 2096 people >65 years of age. The causes of the associated anaemia were determined on laboratory data alone, and therefore may not reflect the true underlying cause. These data are shown in Figure 13.1.

Roughly one-third could be ascribed to a nutritional cause (iron, B_{12} or folate deficiency), one-third to chronic kidney disease and other chronic disorders, and one-third 'unexplained' by other laboratory results. Many of these unexplained anaemias had neutropenia, thrombocytopenia or macrocytosis, which may suggest a myelodysplastic syndrome (MDS) as an underlying aetiology (see later).

ABC of Clinical Haematology, Fourth Edition. Edited by Drew Provan.
© 2018 John Wiley & Sons Ltd. Published 2018 by John Wiley & Sons Ltd.

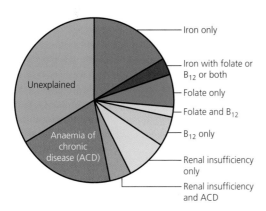

Figure 13.1 Causes of anaemia in older patients, as found in NHANES III study.

Subsequent studies of older adults that examined the causes of anaemia in greater detail suggest that haematological malignancies such as MDS may be common as a cause of anaemia in this age group, and unappreciated anaemia of chronic disease or defective erythropoietin response is also more prevalent than might be expected from studies of laboratory values alone. Often, multiple causes for anaemia may coexist.

Iron deficiency

The investigation and treatment of iron deficiency is covered elsewhere, but there are particular considerations in the older patient. The anaemia is typically associated with a low mean cell volume (MCV), low ferritin and transferrin saturation. However, because of co-morbidities that may increase ferritin as an acute-phase reactant, a ferritin level of 50 μg/L has been suggested to be a more useful threshold for iron deficiency in hospitalised older adults. More specialised tests, such as soluble transferrin receptor–ferritin index, have yet to find their place in routine practice. The gold standard for establishing iron stores is a bone marrow aspirate, but this is a painfully invasive test. A more pragmatic approach if iron deficiency is suspected and laboratory tests are unhelpful is to administer a therapeutic trial of oral iron and look for a rise in reticulocyte count and Hb over the following weeks.

As always, it is important to establish the cause of iron deficiency, once confirmed. Older patients have a high incidence of gastrointestinal (GI) malignancies as a potential source of bleeding. In hospitalised patients >65 years and ferritin <50 μg/L:

- 50% have upper GI lesion
- 25% have lower GI lesion.

Absence of iron deficiency does not exclude GI cancer. Treatment may also be more complicated as oral iron formulations may have prominent side effects in older people. Coexistent renal impairment or inflammation will also blunt the response to iron supplementation.

Megaloblastic anaemia

Megaloblastic anaemia typically presents with high MCV and is well described elsewhere, but there are a few points to be made in the context of older adults. Folate deficiency in this age group may be caused by poor nutrition, alcohol abuse, increased requirements due to disease (e.g. haemolysis or psoriasis) or drugs.

B_{12} deficiency may exist in 10–24% of people >65 years. Commoner causes in this age group include:

- food cobalamin malabsorption
- pernicious anaemia
- gastrectomy and gastritis
- *Helicobacter pylori*
- alcohol abuse.

It is important to look for any associated neurological damage.

Diagnosis is standard: low serum B_{12}/folate. Borderline cases may be confirmed with studies of red cell folate, homocysteine or methylmalonic acid levels. Pernicious-anaemia-associated autoantibodies should be sought in B_{12} deficiency:

- anti-intrinsic factor – 100% specific, 50–70% sensitive;
- anti-gastric parietal cell – more sensitive, less specific.

Anaemia of chronic disease

Owing to the high incidence of co-morbidities in older adults, anaemia of chronic disease (ACD, also known as anaemia of inflammation) is common. Usually associated with infectious, inflammatory or neoplastic disease, ACD can be seen in a variety of conditions, including severe trauma, diabetes mellitus and in those with acute or chronic immune activation.

The anaemia is usually normochromic and normocytic, though a low MCV may also be seen. The aetiology is multifactorial. Abnormal iron metabolism results in reduced iron absorption from the GI tract and iron trapping within macrophages. Erythropoietin levels are often not elevated due to failure of production; and even when levels are high, the response to erythropoietin is blunted. The underlying causes are thought to involve inflammatory cytokines such as interleukin 1 and 6 and tumour necrosis factor alpha. These cytokines are released in a variety of chronic inflammatory states and have multiple effects. One important action is causing a rise in serum levels of the acute-phase protein hepcidin. Hepcidin is released by the liver and appears to act as a master regulator of iron metabolism, though the effects are complex. Assays for elevated hepcidin in the context of ACD have not yet found their place, but research is ongoing.

Ferritin levels are usually elevated, and transferrin saturation is typically normal or low normal. It is often difficult to diagnose ACD, and other causes for anaemia may coexist. The gold standard of evaluating bone marrow iron stores is invasive and generally not used. ACD is typically mild, and blood transfusion is usually not required. The treatment is that of the underlying disorder where possible. Measurement of serum erythropoietin may be helpful, as some patients with low levels may respond to erythropoietin treatment.

Haematological malignancies

As with many other cancers, the incidence of haematological malignancies increases with age. Some malignancies, such as acute lymphoblastic leukaemia and Hodgkin lymphoma, have an incidence peak in childhood or early adulthood; however, the incidence of most other blood cancers increases with age. The incidence rates for most common haematological cancers are shown in Figure 13.2.

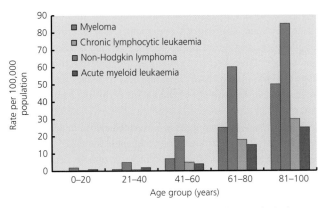

Figure 13.2 The incidence of the four most common haematological malignancies in adults (National Cancer Registration and Analysis Service statistics).

A few specific conditions are discussed because of particular considerations in older adults.

Chronic lymphocytic leukaemia

Chronic lymphocytic leukaemia (CLL) is the most common leukaemia in adults. Approximately half of cases are detected incidentally, because of a full blood count performed for another reason. Unexpected lymphocytosis can be investigated further with blood film and flow cytometric immunophenotyping. Flow cytometry is a very sensitive technique, and it has been shown that routine flow cytometry will detect CLL-like cells in 5% of otherwise healthy individuals >60 years of age. Using highly sensitive techniques in a research setting, low-level CLL cells can be detected in the majority of people >60 years of age. This condition is called monoclonal B-cell lymphocytosis, and most people will never have symptoms ascribable to these low-level clones. Fewer than 1% will progress to overt CLL. It is important to be aware of this relatively common disorder in older adults, as it is likely to cause anxiety if described as leukaemia.

The need for treatment of CLL is based on the presence of symptoms due to lymphadenopathy, night sweats or weight loss, or evidence of bone marrow suppression: anaemia or thrombocytopenia. One-third of people with CLL will never need treatment, but will be regularly followed in outpatient clinics. New models of outpatient follow-up include posting blood samples taken locally to diagnostic centres, Skype clinics and email consultations. Moving care away from tertiary centres into the community may be helpful for older adults who find travel difficult.

Monoclonal gammopathy of undetermined significance

Monoclonal gammopathy of undetermined significance (MGUS) is the asymptomatic precursor to plasma cell (multiple) myeloma. It is analogous to monoclonal B-cell lymphocytosis and is similarly common (see Table 13.1).

In MGUS, a low-level paraprotein is typically detected incidentally. More important than the actual level of the paraprotein is absence of end-organ damage attributable to myeloma:
• hypercalcaemia
• renal failure

Table 13.1 Prevalence of paraproteinaemia in different age groups.

Age (years)	Paraprotein prevalence (%)
≥50 to <70	3.2
≥70 to <85	5.3
≥85	7.5

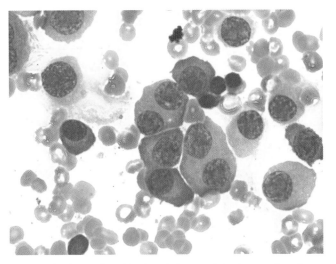

Figure 13.3 Abnormal, multinucleated plasma cells in plasma cell myeloma.

• anaemia
• bone lesions
• amyloidosis.

People with MGUS generally require regular follow-up to monitor for signs of development of myeloma (Figure 13.3), which may develop at a rate of 1% per year.

Myelodysplastic syndromes

The MDSs comprise a heterogeneous group of malignant haematopoietic stem cell disorders characterised by ineffective blood cell production and a variable risk of transformation to acute leukaemia. Patients typically have anaemia, thrombocytopenia, neutropenia or an unexplained macrocytosis. Often, they may be asymptomatic, but symptoms may occur due to these cytopenias or progression to acute leukaemia. The incidence of MDSs rises steeply with age.

The diagnosis of an MDS relies on careful examination of a blood film (Figure 13.4), bone marrow aspirate and cytogenetic studies. Effective treatments for symptomatic MDSs are few and are often limited to supportive care, such as transfusion. Because many patients with suspected MDSs are asymptomatic, conclusive diagnosis may not be made as it requires invasive tests that may not alter management. The true incidence of MDSs in the elderly is therefore underestimated, but studies suggest that up to 25% of unexplained anaemia may be due to an MDS.

Investigation and treatment of suspected haematological malignancies in older people

Beyond the recognition of specific common haematological malignancies, there are some general points to be made about blood cancers in older people. Some of the following findings

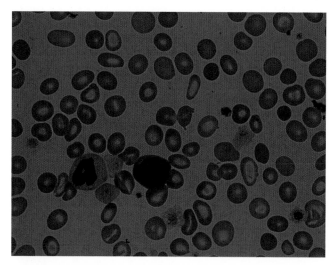

Figure 13.4 Blood film in a patient with an MDS. Shown are giant platelets, a dysplastic neutrophil and a myeloblast.

may flag up a potential haematological malignancy, though these are non-specific:

- night sweats
- bone pain
- weight loss
- hepatosplenomegaly
- lymphadenopathy
- leucopenia
- leucocytosis
- thrombocytopenia
- unexplained macrocytosis
- renal failure.

If there is any suspicion of a haematological malignancy, discussion and possible urgent referral to haematology is recommended.

Haematological malignancies in older adults may present particular treatment challenges. Greater leukaemia mutational genetic complexity is commoner as age increases, which is associated with a more aggressive disease course. The presence of co-morbidities often limits the intensity of treatment and increases the frequency of side effects. Treatment may be aimed at disease control or palliation, rather than cure. Nonetheless, this is a rapidly evolving field, and newer agents are being constantly developed. The needs of older patients with haematological malignancies will expand as the population rises and more therapeutic options become available. A multidisciplinary focus and coordinated, integrated care are required to care for older adults who may have multiple co-morbidities as well as a primary blood condition.

Further reading

Almeida J, Nieto WG, Teodosio C *et al.* (2011) CLL-like B-lymphocytes are systematically present at very low numbers in peripheral blood of healthy adults. *Leukemia*, **25**(4), 718–722.

Bird JM, Owen RG, D'Sa S, *et al.* (2014) Guidelines for the diagnosis and management of multiple myeloma 2011. *British Journal of Haematology*, **154**(1), 32–75.

Cheng CK, Chan J, Cembrowski GS, van Assendelft OW (2004) Complete blood count reference interval diagrams derived from NHANES III: stratification by age, sex, and race. *Laboratory Hematology*, **10**(1), 42–53.

Guralnik JM, Eisenstaedt RS, Ferrucci L, *et al.* (2004) Prevalence of anemia in persons 65 years and older in the United States: evidence for a high rate of unexplained anemia. *Blood*, **104**(8), 2263–2268.

Hassan M, Abedi-Valugerdi M (2014) Hematologic malignancies in elderly patients. *Haematologica*, **99**(7), 1124–1127.

National Cancer National Cancer Registration and Analysis Service (n.d.) Cancer statistics in haematological cancer. www.ncin.org.uk (accessed 10 September 2017).

Stauder R, Thein SL (2014) Anemia in the elderly: clinical implications and new therapeutic concepts. *Haematologica*, **99**(7), 1127–1130.

CHAPTER 14

Haematological Emergencies

Igor Novitzky-Basso[1] and Jim Murray[2]

[1] Queen Elizabeth University Hospital Glasgow, NHS Greater Glasgow and Clyde, Glasgow, UK
[2] University Hospitals Birmingham NHS Foundation Trust, Queen Elizabeth Hospital, Queen Elizabeth Medical Centre, Birmingham, UK

OVERVIEW

- Haematological emergencies require prompt recognition for prompt treatment.
- Spinal cord compression may be the presenting feature in myeloma.
- Platelet transfusions may be lifesaving in disseminated intravascular coagulation.
- Platelet transfusions should be avoided in thrombotic thrombocytopenic purpura.
- Accurate diagnosis of thrombotic thrombocytopenic purpura is crucial to ensure appropriate management.

The importance of the prompt treatment of severe neutropenic sepsis in patients receiving chemotherapy for the treatment of malignant disease is now well recognised. Life-threatening complications such as disseminated intravascular coagulation (DIC) or spinal cord compression may present to the general physician in a variety of clinical circumstances, and prompt recognition of the underlying pathology is crucial for successful management.

Hyperviscosity syndrome

This may result from a number of haematological conditions (Box 14.1). Whole-blood viscosity is a function of the concentration and composition of its components, but is also very dependent upon flow rates. Blood viscosity will be increased by an elevation in the

---

Box 14.1 **Causes of hyperviscosity.**

- Waldenström's macroglobulinaemia
- Acute leukaemia with hyperleucocytosis (white cell count >100 × 10⁹/L, particularly in myeloid leukaemias)
- Polycythaemia vera
- Myeloma

---

cellular constituents (Figure 14.1) (e.g. white blood cells in acute leukaemia and red cells in polycythaemia) or by an increase in plasma proteins (e.g. a monoclonal immunoglobulin in myeloma or lymphoma). The higher viscosity in small vessels leads to sluggish capillary blood flow, which is responsible for the clinical features.

Signs and symptoms of hyperviscosity include neurological disturbance, retinopathy (Figure 14.2) and spontaneous bleeding, usually epistaxis (Table 14.1). The severity of the clinical picture will depend on the characteristics of the cell type or protein that is increased, and will also reflect the level of physiological compensation. Patients with chronic disorders such as polycythaemia vera often only complain of mild headaches, whereas patients with acute leukaemia, notably acute myeloid leukaemias, may present *in extremis*, with marked hypoxia from pulmonary leucostasis, together with altered consciousness and a variety of neurological signs related to reduced cerebral blood flow. Hyperviscosity may also precipitate cardiac failure in susceptible patients.

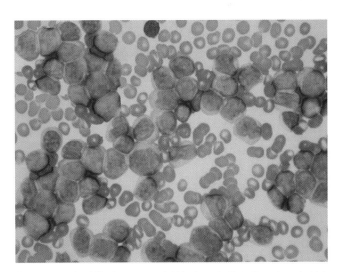

Figure 14.1 Blood film in acute myeloid leukaemia. Note the extremely high number of circulating white blood cells (hyperleucocytosis), leading to hyperviscosity. Source: From Karen Goddard.

ABC of Clinical Haematology, Fourth Edition. Edited by Drew Provan.
© 2018 John Wiley & Sons Ltd. Published 2018 by John Wiley & Sons Ltd.

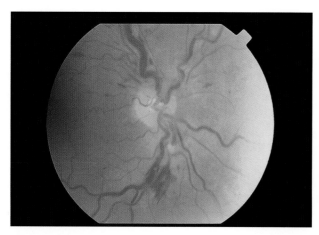 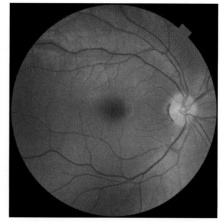

Figure 14.2 Fundal changes in a patient with hyperviscosity (newly diagnosed myeloma) with immunoglogulin (Ig)A concentration 50 g/dL showing retinal venous engorgement, papilloedema and haemorrhages (left) compared with normal (right).

Table 14.1 Symptoms and signs of hyperviscosity.

Symptom	Sign
Headache	
Neurological disturbance	Changes in mental state
	Confusion
	Coma
Ocular disturbance	Dilatation and segmentation of retinal veins
Bleeding	Epistaxis

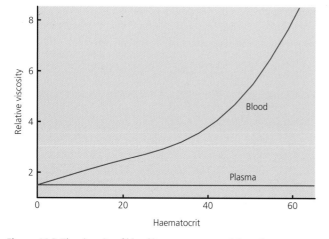

Figure 14.3 The viscosity of blood increases exponentially as the haematocrit rises beyond 45%.

The definitive management of hyperviscosity is through treatment of the underlying condition, usually with chemotherapy. Prompt treatment is needed in severe cases to prevent permanent deficits. For patients presenting with acute leukaemias, leukapheresis may be used as an interim measure until the chemotherapy exerts its full effect. Vigorous hydration and uricosuric agents (rasburicase) are also indicated. For patients with hyperviscosity due to elevated Igs (often IgM or IgA), plasmapheresis is effective in reducing the paraprotein concentration. This may be necessary at disease presentation, but can also be performed at regular intervals

Table 14.2 Sickle cell crises.

Type	Affected area/causes	Symptoms
Commonly		
Vaso-occlusive: can affect any tissue	Bones	Dactylitis
	Abdomen	Splenic infarcts
	Chest	Cerebral infarcts
		Pleuritic pain, may develop into 'chest syndrome', which is associated with progressive respiratory failure
Rarely		
Aplastic	Due to parvovirus B19 infection	
Sequestration	Due to pooling of red cells in spleen or other organs	
Haemolytic	Due to a further reduction in the red cell lifespan	

in symptomatic patients with chemotherapy refractory disease. For patients with polycythaemia (Figure 14.3), isovolaemic venesection will reduce the blood viscosity.

Sickle cell crisis

The sickling disorders result from the inheritance of structural haemoglobin (Hb) variants. Homozygous sickle cell anaemia (Hb SS) is the most common and severe form of sickle cell anaemia in the UK. The compound heterozygotes comprising Hb S in association with Hb C (Hb SC), β thalassaemia (Hb S/β thal) or Hb D (Hb SD) account for the majority of the remaining cases.

Recurrent episodes of acute, severe pain due to vaso-occlusive sickle cell crises are the hallmark of these diseases (Table 14.2). Crises can also result from marrow aplasia, splenic or hepatic sequestration and episodes of haemolysis. The chest syndrome and the girdle syndrome are more severe forms of crisis associated with higher morbidity and mortality (Figure 14.4). Other complications include leg ulcers, renal impairment and retinopathy (Hb SS), and thrombosis (Hb SC).

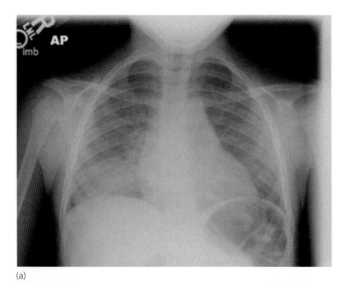

(a)

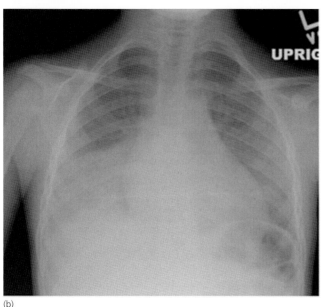

(b)

Figure 14.4 Sickle cell disease. Anteroposterior chest radiographs: (a) at presentation showing generalised air space change/consolidation in the lower zone of the right lung; (b) showing progressive air space changes in the right lower zone a day following presentation. Source: S Yale, N Nagib, and T Guthrie. Acute chest syndrome in sickle cell disease: crucial considerations in adolescents and adults. *Postgraduate Medicine*, Vol 107:No. 1:Jan 2000. Reproduced with permission of Taylor & Francis.

Dehydration, infection, stress or skin cooling may precipitate vaso-occlusive crises. Sickling of the red cells occurs in the small vessels, resulting in decreased tissue blood flow and hypoxia and acidosis, which in turn precipitate further sickling (Figure 14.5).

The aim of treatment is to break this cycle of sickling (Box 14.2). Management, therefore, includes the maintenance of a high fluid intake (60 mL/kg per 24 h) to prevent dehydration and oxygen therapy if hypoxia is confirmed on pulse oximetry. Imperative to the management of patients with sickle cell crises is adequate pain relief. This often requires opiates, given as continuous intravenous or subcutaneous infusions. Sickle cell patients are functionally

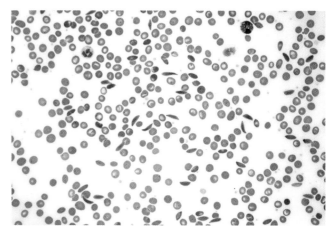

Figure 14.5 Sickled red cells (crescent shaped) in homozygous sickle cell disease. Source: © Visuals Unlimited, Inc. / Dr Gladden Willis, Gettyimages.

Box 14.2 **Treatment of sickle cell crises.**

- Adequate analgesia; usually will require opiates
- Vigorous intravenous hydration
- Oxygen, if hypoxaemic
- Broad-spectrum antibiotics, if signs of infection
- Consider top-up transfusions if Hb has fallen >20 g/L
- Consider exchange transfusion for the chest syndrome, stroke or multi-organ failure

---

asplenic, and broad-spectrum antibiotics should be started in any patient in whom infection is suspected.

Top-up blood transfusions are often unnecessary and should be reserved for patients with signs or symptoms attributable to anaemia, typically when the Hb has fallen more than 20 g/L and is <50 g/L. Transfused red cell products should be matched for Rh (C, D and E) and Kell antigens. Exchange transfusions aim to reduce the level of Hb S to <30% and are indicated in patients with severe chest syndrome, suspected cerebrovascular events, priapism or multi-organ failure. Any patient requiring an exchange transfusion should be discussed with a haematologist.

Spinal cord compression

Patients with haematological disease may present with spinal cord compression. This may be due to tumour deposits, such as lymphoma or plasmacytoma, or a consequence of spinal instability from lytic bone disease in multiple myeloma. Most patients with cord compression complain of pain, which is constant and can be easily confused with degenerative disease. Commonly, signs consistent with root compression, with pain in the affected dermatome, precede the overt signs of cord compression.

The neurological signs accompanying cord compression vary according to both the rapidity of the development of compression and the area of the cord affected (Box 14.3). Acute lesions often result in hypotonia and weakness, whereas chronic lesions are more often associated with the classic upper motor neurone signs of hypertonia and hyper-reflexia. The site of the lesion defines the associated sensory loss, and hyperaesthesia may be seen in the dermatome at the level of the lesion. More lateral lesions may result in dissociated sensory loss (i.e. ipsilateral loss of joint position sense), and proprioception with contralateral loss of pain and temperature. Bladder and bowel disturbances often occur late, with the exception of the cauda equina compression syndrome, in which they are an early feature.

If cord compression is suspected, the definitive investigation is an urgent magnetic resonance scan (Figure 14.6) to establish the presence of cord compression, to delineate the level of the lesion and to plan further treatment. Plain spinal X-rays are useful if myeloma is suspected to demonstrate lytic lesions.

In the acute presentation, high-dose dexamethasone (e.g. 4 mg four times daily) is given. In a patient presenting *de novo* with cord compression, investigations are aimed at establishing an underlying diagnosis, and will usually include protein electro-

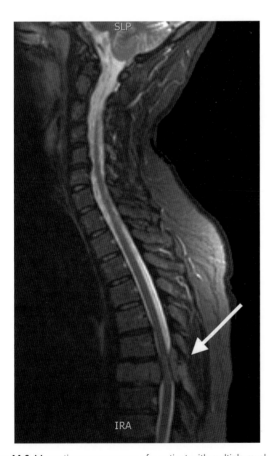

Figure 14.6 Magnetic resonance scan of a patient with multiple myeloma showing loss of height of T7 vertebra with associated spinal cord compression.

phoresis, measurement of tumour markers, including prostate-specific antigen, imaging such as a chest X-ray and/or computed tomography scans, and a tissue biopsy of the lesion to establish the histology. Further management will then depend on the underlying cause, and will often involve a combination of chemotherapy and radiotherapy.

Bleeding

Acute bleeding from trauma or as part of a systemic illness is a frequent cause for attendance to the accident and emergency department. Defects in different phases of haemostasis may lead to uncontrolled bleeding and require specific treatment (Table 14.3).

Anticoagulation

Numerous medical conditions necessitate the use of anticoagulation in order to prevent further thrombosis and consequential increased illness and disability. The most common anticoagulant in use is warfarin, and this is associated with a 1% annual risk of severe (life-threatening) bleeding, requiring complete reversal within 6–7 h. Correction is most effectively and rapidly achieved (within 10 min) by the administration of 25–50 units/kg of prothrombin complex concentrates (PCC), which contain factors II, VII, IX and X. Reversal of warfarin-induced anticoagulation occurs within 10 min of administration, and 5 mg intravenous vitamin K should be given concurrently as some factors in the PCC (factor VII) have a half-life of 6 h. Patients presenting with non-life-threatening bleeding should receive 1–3 mg intravenous vitamin K.

Occasionally, patients may present without bleeding yet have a prolonged international normalised ratio (INR), which puts them at significant risk of severe bleeding. For those with INR >8, 1–5 mg of oral vitamin K is recommended and one or two doses of warfarin withheld, while those with INR between 5 and 8 should have warfarin withheld and their maintenance dose reduced. All patients on warfarin presenting with INR >5 should be investigated for underlying causes.

Novel anticoagulants, such as direct thrombin inhibitors (e.g. dabigatran) or anti-X inhibitors (rivaroxaban) have been shown to have a safety profile equivalent to warfarin, and do not require monitoring of anticoagulant effect. Reversal of anticoagulation in patients with severe bleeding taking novel anticoagulants is difficult as there are no antidotes available, although these are currently in development. Anti-X inhibitors may be reversed partially by the

Table 14.3 Causes of bleeding according to phase of haemostasis.

Phase of haemostasis	Defect
Platelet plug	Low platelet count
	von Willebrand disease
	Defect in platelet function (inherited or due to drugs)
Fibrin clot	Vitamin K deficiency
	Anticoagulation
	Liver disease
	DIC
	Inherited bleeding disorders

use of PCC. For direct thrombin inhibitors there is no effective reversal agent, although dialysis may be effective.

Thrombocytopenia

Modest to moderate reduction in platelet count is not associated with spontaneous haemorrhage, although bleeding following trauma or surgery may be more extensive. Platelet counts of less than 10×10^9/L may be associated with significant bleeding in the context of trivial trauma. Bleeding typically occurs in mucosal surfaces. Common causes of severe thrombocytopenia include immune thrombocytopenic purpura, DIC, consumption due to major haemorrhage or transfusion, liver disease, vitamin B_{12} or folate deficiency, medication (such as thiazides, alcohol, heparin) and disorders of the bone marrow. Occasionally, viral infections such as infectious mononucleosis will result in a profound thrombocytopenia. Depending on the patient's size, one adult dose of platelet will provide an increment in the platelet count of approximately $(30–40) \times 10^9$/L. A platelet count of 30×10^9/L is considered safe for activities of normal daily life, and for most surgical procedures a platelet count of at least 50×10^9/L is recommended. For life-threatening bleeding, such as gastrointestinal haemorrhage or bleeding into the central nervous system, platelet counts of above 75×10^9/L and 100×10^9/L respectively are recommended.

Defects in platelet function

A qualitative defect in platelet function should be considered in a bleeding patient in the absence of von Willebrand disease or low platelet counts. The commonest causes are medical conditions affecting platelet function, such as uraemia, and liver disease, and drugs. Aspirin irreversibly inhibits cyclo-oxygenase-1 (COX-1) and consequently thromboxane production, and is associated with a 1–2% major bleeding risk and up to 10% minor bleeding risk. A dose of 300 mg aspirin will lead to an antiplatelet effect lasting up to 7 days. Clopidogrel, an irreversible inhibitor of the P2Y12 platelet receptor, leads to similar inhibition of platelet function for 5–7 days after the final dose. Non-steroidal anti-inflammatory drugs (NSAIDs), such as ibuprofen, will reversibly inhibit COX-1, and platelet function normalises 24 h following the final dose. In addition, prolonged NSAID use is associated with gastric ulceration. Bleeding is exacerbated in patients taking both antiplatelet agents and anticoagulants such as warfarin, and can be problematic in patients with myeloproliferative disorders treated with aspirin.

In patients with bleeding associated with defects in platelet function, platelet transfusions are usually effective, and muco-cutaneous bleeding may be treated using an antifibrinolytic agent such as tranexamic acid.

Inherited defects in platelet function are rare, and significant bleeding may be treated with desmopressin or platelet transfusions in the case of Glanzmann thrombasthaenia. In most of these disorders minor muco-cutaneous bleeding will respond to antifibrinolytic agents.

Disseminated intravascular coagulation

DIC describes the syndrome of widespread intravascular coagulation induced by blood procoagulants either introduced into or produced in the bloodstream (Table 14.4). These coagulant proteins overcome the normal physiological anticoagulant mechanisms.

Table 14.4 Clinical features of DIC.

Disorder	Features
Bleeding	Spontaneous bruising and petechiae
	Prolonged bleeding from venepuncture sites
	Epistaxis
	Gastrointestinal bleeding
	Pulmonary haemorrhage
	Intracerebral bleed
Thrombosis	Venous thromboembolism
	Skin necrosis
	Acute renal failure (ischaemia of the renal cortex)
	Cerebral infarction
Features related to the underlying disorder	Shock

Table 14.5 Essential diagnostic investigations for DIC.

Investigation	Positive result
Full blood count	Reduced platelet count
Prothrombin time	Increased
Activated partial thromboplastin time	Increased
Fibrinogen	Decreased
D-dimers	Increased

Table 14.6 Causes of acute DIC.

Type	Cause
Infection	Gram-negative infections, endotoxic shock
Obstetric	Placental abruption, intra-uterine death, severe preeclampsia or eclampsia, amniotic fluid embolism
Trauma	Head injury, burns
Malignancy	Carcinoma of the prostate, ovary, colon, pancreas; acute promyelocytic leukaemia
Vascular	Aortic aneurysm, giant haemangioma
Miscellaneous	Transfusion with ABO incompatible blood, hypothermia, drug reactions

The overall result, irrespective of the cause, is widespread tissue ischaemia (due to clot formation, thrombi) and bleeding (due to consumption of clotting factors, platelets, and the production of breakdown products that further inhibit the coagulation pathway).

If the diagnosis of DIC is suspected clinically, investigations should include a full blood count, clotting profile, fibrinogen level and D-dimers (Table 14.5). In DIC, the platelet count is decreased, prothrombin and activated partial thromboplastin times elevated, fibrinogen level decreased and D-dimers increased.

Treatment is primarily directed at the underlying cause (Table 14.6); for example, antibiotics for infection, the removal of the fetus or placenta in cases of retained dead fetus syndrome or placental abruption, or treatment with chemotherapy for acute promyelocytic leukaemia. DIC generally resolves fairly quickly after removal of the underlying cause in obstetric cases, but control of septicaemia can take some time.

Interim supportive measures include intravenous hydration, oxygen therapy and correction of the coagulopathy. Platelet

Box 14.4 **Initial management of DIC**

- Treat as for severe bleeding/shock
- Administer platelets, if platelet count < 50 × 10⁹/L
- Administer fresh frozen plasma to correct prothrombin time and activated partial thromboplastin time
- Administer cryoprecipitate, if fibrinogen is < 1.0 g/L
- Remove/treat the underlying cause

transfusions are generally indicated when the count is <50 × 10⁹/L, fresh frozen plasma to replace clotting factors when the INR or activated partial thrombin ratio is >1.5, and cryoprecipitate when the fibrinogen level is <1.0 g/L (Box 14.4). The use of intravenous heparin is generally contraindicated. The clinical circumstances in DIC can alter very rapidly, and so frequent and serial laboratory monitoring is key to the management.

Thrombotic thrombocytopenic purpura

Thrombotic thrombocytopenic purpura (TTP) is a rare clinical diagnosis characterised by the classic pentad of features, namely thrombocytopenia (Figure 14.7), microangiopathic haemolytic anaemia, fluctuating neurological signs, renal impairment and fever. However, up to 35% of patients do not have neurological symptoms or signs at presentation, and the diagnosis of TTP should be suspected in any patient presenting with a microangiopathic haemolytic anaemia and thrombocytopenia in the absence of any other identifiable cause (Table 14.7).

The syndrome is characterised by the formation of platelet microvascular thrombi, which primarily affect the renal and cerebral circulations. The principal abnormality is a deficiency in a protease called ADAMTS13, the function of which is to cleave ultra-large von Willebrand factor (ULVWF) multimers. In the absence of this protease, ULVWF multimers persist in the plasma and result in

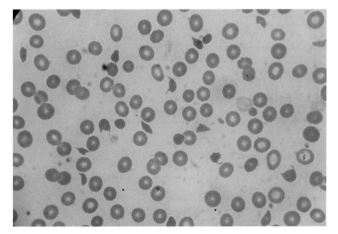

Figure 14.7 Red cell fragments (irregularly shaped cells amongst the normal round red cells) seen on the blood film of a patient with thrombotic thrombocytopenic purpura. Note also the marked thrombocytopenia seen in this blood film. Source: Reproduced with permission from TeamHaem.

Table 14.7 Clinical subtypes of TTP.

Type	TTP subtype	Cause
Congenital		
Acquired	Acute idiopathic	
	Secondary	Drugs: oral contraceptive pill, ticlopidine, ciclosporin, mitomycin C Post-bone-marrow transplantation Systemic lupus erythematosus Malignancy Pregnancy Infection: human immunodeficiency virus, *Escherichia coli* 0157:H7
	Intermittent TTP	Recurrent episodes at unpredictable intervals

spontaneous platelet aggregation in the microcirculation. Congenital, idiopathic and secondary forms of TTP exist.

Historically, in the absence of treatment, the mortality rate of TTP was >90%; however, this has fallen to 10–30% following the institution of urgent plasma exchange for acute TTP. This process both removes the ULVWF multimers from the patient's circulation and replaces the ADAMTS13 protease in the fresh frozen plasma that is used as replacement fluid. Before commencing plasma exchange, a vascular catheter will need to be inserted, but platelet transfusions should be avoided, even in cases with a severe thrombocytopenia, because these patients rarely bleed, and the addition of allogeneic platelets can lead to further platelet aggregation and worsen the underlying condition. Plasma exchange should be continued daily until at least 2 days after the platelet count normalises. If plasma exchange is unavailable, infusions of fresh frozen plasma can be given; however, these are associated with an inferior outcome compared with plasma exchange. Immunosuppressive therapy can reduce synthesis of the abnormal antibodies, and high-dose prednisolone (1 mg/kg) or intravenous methylprednisolone 1 g is started as soon as possible, giving the first dose after plasma exchange. Rituximab (monoclonal anti-CD20 antibody) is given in idiopathic TTP when patients fail to respond to daily plasma exchange and methylprednisolone and has been shown to prevent relapse of the condition.

Infection in patients with impaired immunity

Patients with a variety of haematological diseases are immunocompromised as a result both of their underlying disease and the treatment required for the condition. Impaired immunity to infection may be the result of neutropenia, lymphocytopenia, hypogammaglobulinaemia or a combination of these abnormalities (Table 14.8).

Table 14.8 Risks of infection in patients with no spleen or hypofunctioning spleen.

Incidence	Organisms
Commonly with encapsulated organisms	*Streptococcus pneumoniae* (60%), *Haemophilus influenzae* type b, *Neisseria meningitidis*
Less commonly	*Escherichia coli*, malaria, babesiosis, *Capnocytophaga canimorsus*

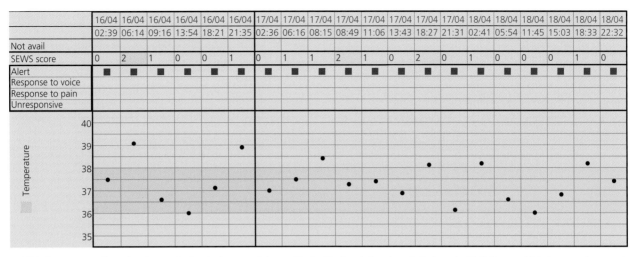

Figure 14.8 Temperature chart showing marked swinging pyrexia in a patient with chronic lymphocytic leukaemia (CLL). Fevers of this type are also seen in other immunocompromised patients, such as those with neutropenia.

A number of haematology patients will be severely neutropenic following either inpatient or outpatient aggressive chemotherapy regimens or as a result of their underlying disease. It is essential that these patients are counselled and supplied with contact numbers and that they understand the urgent need for hospital admission if they become unwell and/or develop a fever. Many of these patients have indwelling tunnelled intravenous catheters, and line-related infections with Gram-positive organisms are common. On admission, all neutropenic patients with a fever (Figure 14.8) or other features of infection should be treated within 1 h with broad-spectrum antibiotics according to the local hospital protocols, which will reflect both the spectrum of causative organisms and their local sensitivities. Removal of the tunnelled catheter may be necessary for severe or persistent line-associated infections.

Patients with CLL often have recurrent infection in the absence of neutropenia, due to the hypogammaglobulinaemia seen in this disorder. Frequent courses of antibiotics may be required, and intravenous immunoglobulins are increasingly being used. Recurrent and severe herpes zoster infections may also occur, and prompt treatment with aciclovir should be given at the first suspicion of herpetic lesions developing. Treatment of CLL may involve purine analogues, such as fludarabine, or the monoclonal antibody alemtuzumab (CamPath®; Genzyme). These both impair T-cell function, rendering the patient at risk of *Pneumocystis jirovecii* (previously known as *Pneumocystis carinii*) pneumonia or cytomegalovirus reactivation. Pneumocystis prophylaxis with co-trimoxazole is initiated coincidentally with treatment with these drugs, and polymerase chain reaction monitoring for cytomegalovirus should be undertaken.

Patients with either functional or anatomical asplenia are at an increased risk of infection with encapsulated organisms, notably *S. pneumoniae*. It is now recommended that all such patients should be vaccinated against *S. pneumoniae*, *H. influenzae* and meningococcus, and remain on lifelong prophylactic antibiotics; for example, penicillin V (Box 14.5). Counselling regarding the need for prompt treatment with antibiotics in the event of a fever is important, and patients should be supplied with an information alert card.

Box 14.5 Recommendations for patients with no spleen or hypofunctioning spleen.

The following vaccinations should be given, ideally 2 weeks before, but alternatively as soon as possible after, splenectomy:

- Pneumococcal vaccine (Pneumovax II) (reimmunise every 5 years)
- *H. influenzae* type b (Hib) vaccine
- Meningococcal polysaccharide vaccine for *N. meningitidis* types A and C
- Influenza B vaccine annually

All patients should receive lifelong prophylaxis with penicillin V (250 mg twice daily) or erythromycin if penicillin allergic

Further reading

British Committee for Standards in Haematology, Blood Transfusion Task Force (2003) Guidelines for the use of platelet transfusions. *British Journal of Haematology*, **122**, 10–23.

Davies JM, Lewis MP, Wimperis J et al. (2011) Review of guidelines for the prevention and treatment of infection in patients with an absent or dysfunctional spleen: prepared on behalf of the British Committee for Standards in Haematology by a working party of the Haemato-Oncology Task Force. *British Journal of Haematology*, **155**, 308–317.

Kyle RA and Disperienzi A (2004) Neurological aspects of monoclonal gammopathy of undetermined significance, multiple myeloma, and related disorders. In *Multiple Myeloma and Related Disorders* (eds G Gahrton, BGM Durie and D Samson), Arnold, London, pp. 350–366.

Oscier D, Dearden C, Eren E et al. (2012) Guidelines on the diagnosis, investigation and management of chronic lymphocytic leukaemia. *British Journal of Haematology*, **159**, 541–564.

O'Shaughnessy DF, Atterbury C, Bolton Maggs P et al. (2004) Guidelines for the use of fresh frozen plasma and cryoprecipitate and cryosupernatant. *British Journal of Haematology*, **126**, 11–28.

Powles R, Sirochi B and Kulkarni S (2003) Investigation and management of hyperleukocytosis in adults. In *The Effective Prevention and Management of Common Complications of Induction Chemotherapy in Haematological Malignancy* (eds R Pinketon, A Rohatiner and A Miles), Aesculapius Medical Press, London, pp. 33–50.

Rees DC, Olujohungbe AD, Parker NE *et al.* (2003) Guidelines for the management of the acute painful crisis in sickle cell disease. *British Journal of Haematology*, **120**, 744–752.

Reinhart WH, Lutolf O, Nydegger U *et al.* (1992) Plasmapheresis for hyperviscosity syndrome in macroglobulinaemia Waldenström and multiple myeloma; influence on blood rheology and the microcirculation. *Journal of Laboratory and Clinical Medicine*, **119**, 69–76.

Scully M, Hunt BJ, Benjamin S *et al.* (2012) Guidelines on the diagnosis and management of thrombotic thrombocytopenic purpura and other thrombotic microangiopathies. *British Journal of Haematology*, **158**, 323–335.

Stone MJ and Bogen SA (2012) Evidence-based focused review of management of hyperviscosity syndrome. *Blood*, **119**, 2205–2208.

Transfusion Task Force (2007) Amendments and corrections to the 'Transfusion Guidelines for neonates and older children' (BCSH, 2004a); and to the ''Guidelines for the use of fresh frozen plasma, cryoprecipitate and cryosupernatant' (BCSH, 2004b). *British Journal of Haematology*, **136**, 514–516.

CHAPTER 15

The Future of Haematology: The Impact of Molecular Biology and Gene Therapy

Katharine Bailey, Richard Burt and Adele K. Fielding

Haematology, Cancer Institute, UCL, Royal Free Campus, London, UK

OVERVIEW

- The techniques of molecular biology, once confined to research laboratories, are increasingly used in diagnosis and monitoring of a wide variety of haematological disorders and will become standard practice.
- Antibodies have found a firm clinical role in the treatment of both malignant and non-malignant haematological disorders. Other 'biological' therapies, such as anti-cancer vaccines and viral vectors for gene therapy, are entering clinical study and are likely to follow suit.
- 'Targeted' drug therapies based on known molecular aberrations will play an increasing role.

Introduction

This chapter will assess the impact of advances in science and technology on the practice of haematology and attempt to predict how haematology might change further over the next 10–15 years (Box 15.1, Table 15.1).

We will focus on several areas of scientific progress and provide specific examples of how the diagnosis or treatment of haematological disorders has benefited from this progress and how it may do so in future.

Gene therapy

'Gene therapy' means introducing genes or genetically modified cells for therapeutic benefit (Table 15.2). Haematological tissues such as bone marrow stem cells or T cells are ideal targets, being readily accessible for manipulation *ex vivo*. Genes are most often delivered by viral vectors, taking advantage of the natural capacity of viruses to act as gene delivery vehicles – retroviruses, lentiviruses, adenoviruses and adeno-associated viruses (AAVs) are most commonly used, but none is without some risk.

Retroviral and lentiviral vectors can stably integrate genes into the chromosome of the host cells, crucial for achieving adequate gene expression in the progeny of the target cells. The first successful clinical

Box 15.1 **The future of haematology: diagnosis and treatment.**

Diagnosis
- More DNA/RNA-based diagnosis, including next-generation sequencing and/or gene profiling for all patients with newly diagnosed haematological malignancies
- Discovery of further molecular abnormalities underlying haematological disorders leading to increased diagnostic precision and more sensitive monitoring of diseases (e.g. minimal residual disease)
- Increased use of molecular monitoring during therapy

Treatment
- New drugs tailored to molecular abnormalities with shift towards totally chemotherapy-free regimens for haematological malignancies
- New biological agents, viruses and viral vectors, monoclonal antibodies (mAbs), chimeric antigen receptors
- Gene therapy – has potential for many haematological disorders, in particular single gene disorders

application of gene therapy was retroviral delivery of the gene encoding adenosine deaminase (ADA) to a patient with ADA-deficient severe combined immunodeficiency in 1990. Subsequently, delivery of a functional interleukin-2 receptor gamma gene generated immune reconstitution in patients with X-linked severe combined immunodeficiency. However, one in three developed T-cell leukaemia due to 'insertional mutagenesis' following activation of the *LMO2* oncogene. The next 10 years is likely to see wider, safer use of gene therapy using lentiviral vectors. The single gene disorders haemophilia A and B are ideal candidates, since small increases in production of the missing coagulation factor can significantly reduce clinical bleeding (Figure 15.1). Recently, stable factor IX expression of 1–6%, consequent on therapeutic expression from an AAV vector was demonstrated in six adult males with severe haemophilia B, four of whom could discontinue factor IX concentrate prophylaxis. Obstacles to success included toxicity of the delivery vector, and immune response to the

ABC of Clinical Haematology, Fourth Edition. Edited by Drew Provan.
© 2018 John Wiley & Sons Ltd. Published 2018 by John Wiley & Sons Ltd.

Table 15.1 Scientific techniques and approaches that will continue to make major contributions to modern haematology

Technique	Applications in haematology
Gene cloning and sequencing allow identification, characterisation and manipulation of genes responsible for specific products or diseases. *Next-generation gene sequencing* (NGS) allows rapid sequencing of large amounts of DNA.	Elucidation of the molecular pathology of disease and diagnostic tests based on the polymerase chain reaction (PCR). Whole exome sequencing enables the discovery of somatic clonal mutations (e.g. *BRAF* V600E in hairy cell leukaemia). There is great potential for discovering mutations in individual patients, moving towards individualised targeted therapy. Gene arrays enable the analysis of patterns of gene regulation in individual patients.
Gene expression profiling enables the measurement of the activity of thousands of genes simultaneously using DNA microarray technology. *PCR* is a highly sensitive and versatile technique for amplifying very small quantities of DNA. Amplification of RNA molecules is possible after initial reverse transcription of RNA into DNA.	Rapid diagnosis of infectious diseases in immunocompromised patients (e.g. hepatitis C, cytogemalovirus reactivations); minimal residual disease detection in haematological malignancies where the molecular defect is known; carrier detection and antenatal diagnosis in haemophilias and hereditary anaemias.
Monoclonal antibodies permit precise diagnosis and, increasingly, therapy.	Increased diagnostic precision, 'positive purging,' *ex vivo* gene delivery, and *ex vivo* expansion of progenitor cells are possible as a result of the fact that populations of haemopoietic cells containing a high proportion of primitive progenitors can be isolated.

Table 15.2 Gene therapy strategies

Strategy	Potential application
Corrective replacement	Sickle cell disease: to replace the point mutation that causes the substitution of valine for glutamine on the sixth amino acid residue of the β globin chain
Corrective gene addition	Haemophilia: to introduce a gene for missing coagulation protein
Pharmacological	Continuous production of interferon alfa, erythropoietin or other therapeutic proteins
Cytotoxic	Leukaemia: targeted delivery of cytotoxic proteins
Prophylactic	Chemoprotection: drug-resistance genes introduced into haemopoietic stem cells, conferring resistant phenotype, thus protecting against chemotherapeutic agents
Replicating virus therapy	Oncolytic viruses may be used to directly kill transformed cells

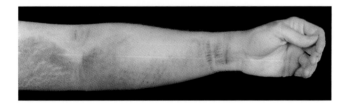

Figure 15.1 Haemophilic patient with inhibitors and severe spontaneous bleeding. Gene therapy approaches can make this a thing of the past.

vector or coagulation factor. A more significant challenge for the next 10 years is the development of gene therapy for haemophilia A, a much more common disorder due to lack of factor VIII, which is a very large protein, so that the gene is hard to package in the AAV vectors used.

Haemoglobinopathies are also being addressed by gene therapy; the first successful gene therapy for transfusion-dependent thalassaemia was achieved in 2007 using a lentiviral vector to transduce stem cells which were reinfused following myeloablative busulphan conditioning. After engraftment the patient had a gradual increase in gene-marked cells to 10–20% and became transfusion independent by 2 years after gene transfer.

Genomics

Genomics is 'the systematic study of all the genes of an organism'. Expression profiling using 'arrays' is one way to study all the genes currently being expressed in a given cell or tissue under defined conditions. Thousands of unique probes are robotically deposited on a 'DNA chip', creating the 'array'. To profile gene expression in the tissue of interest, messenger RNA (mRNA) is isolated, copied into DNA, labelled with a fluorescent dye and then hybridised (stuck) to the chip – complementary DNAs (cDNAs) that are expressed can 'stick' and be detected. In recent years, numerous studies involving microarray-based gene-expression profiling (Figure 15.2) have identified novel prognostic subgroups and enabled prediction of which subgroups of patients will respond to certain treatments – lymphoma is a key example where this work has changed the way we classify patients.

A new class of gene regulation molecule, small non-coding RNAs, termed microRNAs, can degrade target mRNA, thereby affecting post-transcriptional gene expression. MicroRNA gene expression profiles can predict prognosis in chronic lymphocytic leukaemia. The future is likely to see further characterisation of mircoRNA in the diagnoses and treatment of leukaemias.

NGS provides a paradigm shift in the way genetic information is extracted from biological systems. Genomic DNA of interest is fragmented into millions of small segments, which are attached to a scaffold. These small segments are sequenced in millions of parallel reactions. The newly identified sequence of bases, the 'reads', are then reassembled, either using a known reference genome as a scaffold (resequencing) or without a reference genome (*de novo* sequencing). It is now possible to sequence several complete human genomes in a single run, generating data in about 1 week, for approximately $5000 per genome. By contrast, the first human genome sequenced in 2003 took more than 10 years and cost nearly $3 billion. The main limitation to routine use of NGS is the handling of the vast and complex information by bioinformaticians. Despite this, limited NGS is increasingly used in direct clinical care, including for prenatal testing and to identify rare genetic variants in monogenic disorders. In haematological malignancies, efficient detection of

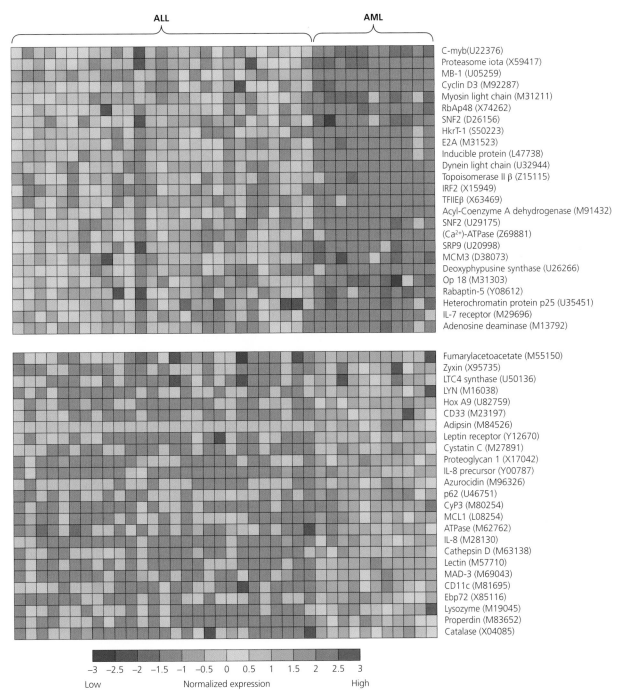

Figure 15.2 Microarray technology allows the analysis of thousands of different genes simultaneously. Reproduced from Aitman (*British Medical Journal* 2001;**323**:611–615) and adapted from Golub TR, Slonim DK, Tamayo P, Huard C, Gaasenbeek M, Mesirov JP, *et al.* Molecular classification of cancer: class discovery and class prediction by gene expression monitoring (*Science* 1999;**286**:531–537).

either inherited or somatic mutations in cancer genes by NGS has contributed to characterising haematological disease by identifying novel driver mutations in a number of different malignancies. It is also beginning to be used for minimal residual disease quantification in these settings. In the future, current challenges of NGS, such as differentiating 'driver mutations' from 'passenger mutations' and evaluating prognostic and predictive value of identified mutations, will be addressed.

Genome editing

Genome editing allows DNA to be inserted, replaced or removed from a genome using artificially engineered nucleases, enzymes that can cleave the phosphodiester bonds between the nucleotide subunits of nucleic acids and hence create double-stranded breaks at desired locations in the genome. 'Cuts' or breaks can be repaired by using a cell's endogenous mechanisms; for example, homologous recombination and nonhomologous end-joining. The likely candidate enzymes for genome editing are zinc finger nucleases, transcription activator-like effector nucleases and the CRISPR/Cas system.

The advantages of this approach over conventional gene therapy approaches are avoidance of insertional mutagenesis and no requirement for long-term expression of a novel gene, since the old genetic defect will be permanently corrected. Once this technology is refined, it will be ideally suited to allow genetic correction of disorders such as sickle cell disease.

Immunological modulation without bone marrow transplant

Monoclonal antibodies

The late 1990s saw the development of rituximab, a humanised chimeric mAb that targets the B-cell marker CD20. It has transformed the treatment of lymphoma and has paved the way for numerous antibody therapies. Their unique mechanisms of action, non-cross resistance and non-additive toxicities make mAbs attractive anticancer therapies. The majority of mAbs target single cellular receptors; however, the next decade or two is likely to see the introduction of therapeutics that can bind multiple targets. The bispecific T-cell engager blinatumumab engages CD3 on cytotoxic T cells and CD19 on malignant B-cells, thus harnessing the patient's own T cells.

Chimeric antigen receptor T cells

There is great interest in engineered T-cell receptors that can be targeted to a tumour-associated antigen; these chimeric antigen receptors are fusions of the single-chain variable fragments of mAbs to the CD3 T-cell receptor. The specificity of patients' own T cells towards cancer targets can be modified *ex vivo* using retroviral vectors. These 'reprogrammed' T cells are cytotoxic to the autologous tumour after reinfusion. Evidence of considerable efficacy is accumulating in early trials in acute lymphoblastic leukaemia. This potent engagement of the patients' immune response comes with immunological effects, particularly related to cytokine release.

Oncolytic viruses

Viruses that preferentially infect and destroy malignant cells whilst leaving normal cells unharmed are increasingly being seen as a future therapeutic option. There are at least nine viruses that have oncolytic properties across a range of malignancies. Amongst haematological malignancies perhaps the most promise has been seen with the vaccine strain of measles virus, which has shown potential for treating myeloma and lymphoma. It can be hidden in carrier cells to avoid a neutralising immune response. These viruses act by recruiting both innate and adaptive immune responses, as well as by direct killing of cancer cells.

Rational drug design

Modulation of epigenetic expression

Epigenetic modifications are reversible modifications that may affect gene expression without altering the DNA sequence; for example, DNA methylation or acetylation of histone proteins.

DNA methylation is often altered within cancer cells. The 'demethylating agents', such as the DNA methyltransferase inhibitor 5-aza-2′-deoxycytidine, can contribute to the treatment of myelodysplastic syndrome, slowing the progression to acute myeloid leukaemia with less toxicity than conventional chemotherapy can. Overexpression of histone deacetylase (HDAC) is common in peripheral T-cell lymphomas and acute myeloid leukaemia and contributes to prevention of apoptosis – HDAC inhibitors can modify this epigenetic regulation to induce apoptosis and prevent growth of the tumour.

Targeting receptor signalling pathways

The development of the Abl-specific tyrosine kinase inhibitor imatinib for the treatment of disorders resulting from *BCR–ABL* translocations was an important paradigm shift in targeted therapy. Underlying molecular abnormalities have been discovered in other malignancies. Janus kinase (JAK)2 is mutated in approximately 97% of patients with the myeloproliferative neoplasm polycythaemia vera; this allows both accurate diagnosis and a novel approach to therapy which also applies to approximately 50% with essential thrombocythaemia and primary myelofibrosis. Ruxolitinib is a JAK inhibitor that is effective in reducing symptoms and spleen size in these disorders. Ibrutinib is an inhibitor of Bruton tyrosine kinase (BTK) an enzyme that is involved in the signal transduction of the B-cell receptor. Activation of BTK normally leads to the activation of cell survival pathways such as nuclear factor-κB (a family of transcription factors known to inhibit tumour necrosis factor-induced apoptosis) and MAP kinases via Src family kinases. Thus, BTK inhibition promotes apoptosis of chronic lymphocytic leukaemia cells and is currently showing promise in clinical trials with efficacy and minimal side effects.

Conclusion

Soon, we will be able to engineer genomes. The explosion of targeted treatments will lead to the introduction of entirely non-chemotherapy regimens for haematological malignancies. The ability to rapidly sequence whole genomes also makes tailoring individual therapies to a patient a possibility. The increasing rationality of our approaches is costly and needs to be accompanied by an increased public understanding of science so that there can be a rational debate about which of these technologies we are willing to pay for and under what circumstances.

Glossary

Apoptosis   A process of programmed cell death.
Epigenetics   Heritable changes in gene expression not produced by a change in DNA sequence.
Genomics   The systematic study of the human genome.
Haemopoietic stem cell   This is a type of post-natal/adult stem cell which is tissue specific. They give rise to all lineages of haemopoietic cells.
HDACs   Histones are proteins that bind to DNA. HDACs are enzymes that catalyse the removal of acetyl groups from histone proteins, thereby affecting and usually increasing gene transcription.

Insertional mutagenesis   A mutation is caused by the introduction of foreign DNA sequences into a gene.

MicroRNA   Small non-coding RNA involved in post-transcriptional gene expression regulation.

Minimal residual disease   Cancer that is still present in the body after treatment but remains undetectable by conventional means (e.g. light microscopy).

Next-generation sequencing (NGS)   Technology enabling rapid sequencing of large quantities of DNA.

Oncogene/tumour suppressor gene   A gene that normally directs cell growth. If altered, can promote or allow the uncontrolled growth of cells and malignant transformation.

PCR   Process by which pieces of DNA can be rapidly and accurately amplified by a method involving thermal cycling.

Reverse transcription   Process by which RNA is used as a template for the production of a DNA copy (cDNA).

Transcription factor   Protein that is able to bind to chromosomal DNA close to a gene and thereby regulates the expression of the gene.

Further reading

Castleton A, Dey A, Beaton B *et al.* (2014) Human mesenchymal stromal cells deliver systemic oncolytic measles virus to treat acute lymphoblastic leukemia in the presence of humoral immunity. *Blood*, **123**(9), 1327–1335.

Dong A, Rivella S and Breda L (2013) Gene therapy for hemoglobinopathies: progress and challenges. *Translational Research*, **161**(4), 293–306.

Meldrum C, Doyle M and Tothill R (2011) Next generation sequencing for cancer diagnostics: a practical perspective. *The Clinical Biochemist Reviews*, **32**(4), 177–195.

Nathwani A, Tuddenham E, Rangarajan S *et al.* (2011) Adenovirus-associated virus vector-mediated gene transfer in haemophilia B. *New England Journal of Medicine*, **365**, 2357–2365.

Patel JP, Gonen M, Figueroa ME *et al.* (2012) Prognostic Relevance of integrated genetic profiling in acute myeloid leukemia. *New England Journal of Medicine*, **366**, 1079–1089.

Qasim W and Thrasher AJ (2014) Progress and prospects for engineered T cell therapies. *British Journal of Haematology*, **166**(6), 818–829.

Index

Note: page numbers in *italics* refer to figures, those in **bold** refer to tables.

ABC of Clinical Haematology, Fourth Edition. Edited by Drew Provan.
© 2018 John Wiley & Sons Ltd. Published 2018 by John Wiley & Sons Ltd.